UNLOCKING YOUR INNER STRENGTH

A Guide to Self-Discovery and Personal Growth

Mujahid Bakht

EBook ISBN: 979-8-89302-056-4

Paperback ISBN: 979-8-89302-054-0

Hardcover ISBN: 979-8-89302-055-7

Published By:

ATLAS AMAZON, LLC.

244 Fifth Avenue, D210, New York, N.Y.

United States of America

SECOND EDITION

TABLE OF CONTENTS

ABOUT THE AUTHOR

LIFE HISTORY: Mr. Bakhtis a mature, experienced, excessively enthusiastic, energetic administrator with thirty-eight years of proven experience as a businessman in international marketing and public relations. Mr. Bakht is an International Real Estate Specialist and Professional Business and Projects Consultant and Advisor. He was born in Pakistan and educated in Pakistan and the USA. Presently, American Citizen belongs to a business-oriented family. Thirty-eight years Resident of New York, USA.

BUSINESS HISTORY: Mr. Bakht is a Founder and President of Atlas Amazon, LLC., Mr. Bakht is a business developer and multilingual business specialist in the Caribbean, South East Asia, and the Middle East emerging markets Mr. Bakht has served, met, and hosted many heads of the States. Also, maintain a close relationship with investors of high net worth in the USA.

CAREER: Mr. Bakht has been engaged with many multinational companies in the fields of international real estate investment, communication, technology, diamond, gold, mining, Pre-Feb housing, wind and solar energy, outsourcing management, and project consulting, along with business partners and associates worldwide. Mr. Bakht has participated in major national and international conferences, including participated in United Nations (U.N.O.) conferences.

TRAVEL: Mr. Bakht is well-traveled and has visited many countries around the world.

MANAGEMENT EXPERIENCE: Thirty-eight years of diversified experience in project consulting, marketing, and business management. As a Director of Marketing, Director of Public Relations, Director of International Affairs, Executive Vice President, President, CEO, and Chairman of many national and multinational companies. Mr. Bakht hired and trained many professionals as business consultants in international marketing and supervised them.

CERTIFICATE OF ACHIEVEMENT: The Achievement Award was presented to Mr. Bakht by Stephen Fossler for five years of continued growth and customer satisfaction from 1996 to 2001.

HONORS MEMBER:Madison Who's Who of Professionals, having demonstrated exemplary achievement and distinguished contributions to the business community, registered at the Library of Congress in Washington D.C. USA. (2007 and 2008)

HONORS MEMBER: Premiere Who's Who International, professional business executive having demonstrated exemplary achievement and distinguished contributions to the International business community, 2008 and 2009.

CERTIFICATES: Certificate of Authenticity from Bill Rodham Clinton, President of the United States, and Hillary Rodham Clinton First Lady, USA. (July 20, 2000);

CERTIFICATE OF AUTHENTICITY: from Terence R. McAuliffe, Chairman of Democratic National Committee, Tom Dachle, Senate Democratic Leader, Dick Gephardt, House Democratic Leader, USA. (June 16, 2001);

CERTIFICATE OF AUTHENTICITY: from Terence R. McAuliffe, Chairman of Democratic National Committee, USA. (April 16, 2002).

INTRODUCTION

Everyone faces challenges in life. Some days feel easy, while others test your patience, courage, and sense of self. In these moments, what helps you keep going is not just your skills or knowledge, but your inner strength? This strength is a quiet power inside each person. It gives you the ability to stand up after failure, move forward during tough times, and stay hopeful when things seem uncertain.

Many people do not realize the strength they already possess. Some believe that confidence, resilience, and self-belief are reserved for a select few exceptional individuals. The truth is that anyone can develop inner strength. It is not about being perfect or never feeling fear. It's about learning how to utilize your resources—your thoughts, feelings, and willpower—to navigate life's ups and downs.

This book is written for you if you want to understand yourself better and become stronger from the inside out. Here, you will find simple and practical ideas and techniques. You don't need any special background to start; you only need an open mind and a willingness to learn about yourself.

The pages ahead will guide you through understanding what inner strength is, why it matters, and how to cultivate it over time. You will learn how to manage self-doubt, set practical goals, recover from setbacks, and develop habits that promote your overall well-being. The goal is to help you feel more in control, more confident, and more at peace with who you are.

Building inner strength is a journey. You do not have to do it all at once. Take each step at your own pace. Celebrate your progress, learn from your mistakes, and keep going. By the end of this book, you will see that you already have what it takes to live a stronger, happier, and more meaningful life.

CHAPTER 1

Understanding Inner Strength

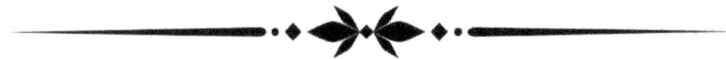

——••◆◆◆••——

Inner strength is something that resides within everyone, but many people never stop to consider what it truly means. It is not about having an authoritarian personality or hiding your emotions. Instead, it is the steady force that helps you handle stress, recover from setbacks, and keep moving forward no matter what life brings.

In this chapter, we will examine inner strength in greater detail. You will learn how it shapes the way you face problems, make decisions, and treat yourself and others. Understanding inner strength is the first step in building a happier, more balanced life. No matter where you start, everyone can discover and grow this strength within themselves.

Defining Inner Strength

Inner strength is the quiet support that helps you get through hard times. It is not always visible to others, but it shows in the way you handle stress, disappointment, or pressure. Unlike physical strength, which is measured by muscles or endurance, inner strength is about your mindset and emotions.

You use inner strength when you face a challenge, but refuse to give up. It is there when you choose to stay calm instead of reacting in anger or panic. Inner strength is also what helps you stand up for your values, even when others disagree with you.

Some people think you are either born with inner strength or you are not. The truth is, everyone has it, and it can grow over time. It manifests in various forms, including patience, hope, honesty, courage, and self-control. Sometimes, you may only notice your inner strength when you look back at difficult moments and realize you managed to persevere.

Inner strength does not mean you never feel sad, scared, or tired. Instead, it helps you move forward, even when you do feel those things. It is the foundation for building confidence, managing stress, and living in a way that aligns with your true self.

The Key Components

Inner strength is not a single quality. It is composed of several key components that work together, enabling you to navigate life's challenges. Understanding these key parts can make it easier to notice and develop them in your own life. Here are some of the main building blocks of inner strength:

Resilience

Resilience is your ability to bounce back after difficulties. Life will always bring unexpected events—some big, some small. A resilient person does not pretend everything is perfect, but they do not stay down for long after a setback. They accept what has happened, learn from it, and look for a way forward. Resilience is what allows you to recover from disappointment, loss, or failure. It grows with practice and experience. Each time you get through a tough time, your resilience becomes a little stronger.

Self-Awareness

Self-awareness means truly understanding yourself—your feelings, thoughts, habits, and triggers. It is paying attention to how you react in different situations. People with good self-awareness can notice when they are feeling stressed or upset before those feelings take over. They understand what motivates them, and they recognize their strengths and weaknesses. This knowledge enables you to make more informed choices and respond to life in a more balanced and effective manner.

Self-Confidence

Self-confidence is the belief in your abilities and the trust in yourself to handle new or difficult situations. It's not about thinking you're perfect or never making mistakes. Instead, it is knowing you can learn and improve. Confident people try new things, set goals, and do not let fear stop them. They accept both praise and criticism without letting either control their sense of worth. Building self-confidence is a lifelong process, but every small success helps it grow and flourish.

Courage

Courage is not the absence of fear; it is taking action despite being afraid. Sometimes, courage means standing up for what is right, speaking your mind, or facing an uncertain future with confidence. Other times, it means admitting when you need help or being honest about your feelings. Courage allows you to take risks, try new things, and grow as a person.

Patience

Patience is the ability to wait without becoming angry or upset. It is helpful in many areas of life, from working towards a goal to interacting with others. Patient people understand that progress takes time and that setbacks are part of any journey. Patience helps you stay calm when things do not go as planned and keeps you from making rushed decisions you might later regret.

Optimism

Optimism is a hopeful and positive outlook on life. It does not mean ignoring problems or pretending everything is fine. Instead, it is believing that even in hard times, good things are possible. Optimistic people look for solutions rather than just focusing on what is wrong. This attitude gives you energy to keep going and helps you find opportunities in difficult situations.

Self-Control

Self-control refers to your ability to manage your impulses, emotions, and behaviors in an effective manner. It helps you stay committed to your goals, make informed decisions, and avoid actions that you might regret. People with strong self-control do not let anger or frustration take over. Instead, they pause, think, and choose their response.

All these qualities—resilience, self-awareness, self-confidence, courage, patience, optimism, and self-control—come together to create your inner strength. You may find that some are stronger in you than others. That is normal. The important thing is to recognize them, appreciate them, and continue working to make them an integral part of your daily life.

Different Types of Inner Strength

Inner strength is a broad concept that encompasses a range of qualities. Each person has a unique blend of strengths that helps them navigate life's demands. Understanding the different types of inner strength can help you notice which ones are already present in your life and which ones you may want to grow.

Emotional Strength

Emotional strength refers to your ability to manage your feelings, particularly during challenging situations. This kind of strength helps you stay calm, even when you are upset or under pressure. People with strong emotional strength can healthily express their emotions and do not let anger or sadness control their actions. They also have compassion for themselves and others.

Mental Strength

Mental strength is your ability to focus, solve problems, and think clearly, even when things are hard. This type of strength helps you push through when you feel like giving up. It enables you to stay on track with your goals and keeps you motivated to keep learning and improving. Mental strength is also about being flexible and able to change your thinking when needed.

Physical Strength

Physical strength is often the first kind we notice, but it encompasses more than just muscles or endurance. Physical strength also involves taking care of your body through regular exercise, adequate sleep, and a balanced diet. When your body is healthy, it supports your mind and emotions, making it easier to face challenges.

Spiritual Strength

Spiritual strength is about finding meaning and purpose in life. This does not have to be connected to religion, although it can be. People with spiritual strength have a sense that their life matters and that they are part of something bigger. This type of strength can give comfort during difficult times and help you feel more hopeful about the future.

Social Strength

Social strength refers to the ability to build and maintain healthy relationships. You can communicate effectively, listen attentively to others, and ask for support when needed. People with strong social skills know how to work effectively with others, handle disagreements constructively, and offer assistance to those around them.

Moral Strength

Moral strength is the courage to stand up for what you believe is right, even when it is not popular or easy. This type of strength enables you to make decisions that align with your values. People with strong moral strength are honest, fair, and willing to take responsibility for their actions.

Creative Strength

Creative strength is your ability to think in innovative ways and devise original solutions. It shows in your willingness to try new things, adapt to change, and look for possibilities instead of problems. Creative strength helps you find opportunities where others might only see challenges.

Comparison of Different Types of Inner Strength

Type of Strength	What It Focuses On	Example in Daily Life
Emotional	Managing feelings	Staying calm during an argument
Mental	Problem-solving, focus	Solving a complex issue at work or school
Physical	Health and body care	Keeping a regular exercise routine
Spiritual	Meaning and purpose	Finding comfort in difficult times
Social	Relationships and teamwork	Reaching out to a friend for support
Moral	Values and integrity	Admitting a mistake and correcting it
Creative	New ideas and solutions	Finding a fresh approach to a problem

Each type of inner strength plays a special role in your life. Together, they help you face challenges, reach your goals, and live in a way that matches your values.

How Inner Strength Is Developed

Inner strength is not something people are just born with—it is something anyone can build, no matter where they start. It grows over time through the choices you make and how you handle the challenges in your life. One crucial way inner strength develops is through learning from difficult experiences. Whenever life gets hard, you have a chance to discover what you are capable of. Even if things do not turn out as you hoped, you can look back, think about what happened, and figure out what you might do differently next time. This process helps you become more prepared for whatever comes in the future.

Taking time to reflect on your thoughts, feelings, and actions also helps your inner strength grow. You might ask yourself how you reacted to a stressful moment or what you learned from a challenging situation. Some people find it helpful to write in a journal, but even a few quiet minutes of thought at the end of the day can make a big difference. The more you understand yourself, the easier it becomes to make wise choices instead of just reacting without thinking.

Building healthy habits is another essential part of developing inner strength. Simple routines like eating well, staying active, getting enough rest, and keeping your space organized may seem basic, but they set the stage for a calmer, more focused mind. Good habits give you energy and support you when life feels overwhelming. Even small, positive changes—done every day—add up over time.

Support from others matters, too. Nobody can face everything alone. Talking with friends, family members, or trusted mentors provides different perspectives, comfort, and encouragement. Letting others know what you're going through does not make you weak; it helps you remember that you're not alone. Sometimes, just knowing someone understands can give you the strength to keep going.

Growth also comes from trying new things and stepping out of your comfort zone. When you learn a new skill or take on a new responsibility, you might feel nervous at first. But each time you face something unfamiliar, you build courage—even if things do not go perfectly. Over time, these small acts of bravery accumulate, increasing your confidence in your abilities.

It is essential to remember that developing inner strength requires time and patience. Some days you may feel strong, and other days you may feel discouraged. This is normal for everyone. Being gentle with yourself and allowing room for mistakes is part of the process. Progress can be slow, but each small step counts.

Learning new things from books, courses, or wise people can help you see situations in a new light. Sometimes, one new idea can change the way you handle a problem. Taking care of your health also plays a significant role. When you get enough sleep, eat nutritious food, and stay active, you feel better overall and are better equipped to face life's ups and downs.

Inner strength does not come all at once. It grows each time you choose to keep going, reflect on what you learn, and try again. Over time, you will notice that challenges no longer feel as overwhelming as they did before. That is the sign that your inner strength is working for you, getting stronger every day.

Benefits of Inner Strength

Having inner strength brings many good changes to your life. When you are strong on the inside, you can handle problems more effectively. Life is never perfect for anyone. Sometimes things go as planned, and at other times, they fall apart. Inner strength is what helps you keep going, even when you feel sad, worried, or confused.

One of the most significant benefits of inner strength is that it enables you to handle stress and challenging situations better. You will still feel upset sometimes, but you can calm yourself down and look for a solution. You do not fall apart or feel lost for a long time. Instead, you face your problems one step at a time. You know that even if things are bad today, they can get better if you keep trying. This helps you worry less and feel more in control.

Inner strength also fosters self-confidence and self-assurance. When you have this kind of strength, you trust your ideas and choices. You do not need others to tell you what to do all the time. You feel confident setting goals for yourself, whether they are big or small. You know you might not always get things right, but you are willing to try. This confidence helps you grow as a person, and it gives you the courage to try new things or face your fears.

Another benefit is that inner strength helps you bounce back from failure or disappointment. Everyone has bad days or makes mistakes. What matters most is how you respond. People with inner strength do not let failure stop them. They learn from it, adjust their plans, and try again. This way, each problem becomes a lesson, rather than a reason to give up.

Having strong inner strength also improves your relationships. When you are strong inside, you can speak honestly about your feelings without fear. You can listen to others, offer sound advice, and provide support to your friends and family. If you need help, please don't hesitate to ask. You can handle arguments or misunderstandings without losing your temper. This fosters more open, healthy, and trusting relationships.

Inner strength helps you stay positive. You can see the good in yourself and others, even during hard times. You do not let negative thoughts take over. When you're feeling low, remind yourself of your strengths or look for things to be grateful for. This positive mindset makes it easier to enjoy life, even when things are not perfect.

Another benefit is that inner strength makes you more independent. You do not always need approval from others. You can decide what is right for you and follow your values. You become better at saying "no" when something does not feel right, and you are less likely to be pressured by others.

Inner strength helps you grow and learn. You are not afraid to make mistakes or try new things. Every challenge you face makes you stronger. Over time, you become wiser and more comfortable with yourself. You learn how to handle different situations, and you feel more at peace in your daily life.

Inner strength enables you to live a happier, more fulfilling life. You become more confident, hopeful, and able to enjoy each day, no matter what happens. This kind of strength is something you can always depend on, and it helps you build the life you truly want.

Common Myths and Misconceptions

When you build up your inner strength, you are giving yourself a gift that continues to help you every single day. Life is full of ups and downs. Sometimes things go your way, and sometimes they do not. What makes the difference is how you handle those challenging moments—and that's where inner strength comes in.

Imagine having a quiet power inside you that helps you stay steady, even when life feels stormy. That is what inner strength does. When things go wrong or you face a setback, you do not just fall apart. You pause, take a breath, and remind yourself that you have been through tough times before — and you made it through. Instead of panicking, you start looking for a way forward, step by step. It is like having an anchor in your heart that keeps you from drifting away in the middle of a storm.

Inner strength also helps you believe in yourself, even when nobody else is watching. You start to trust your own decisions, big or small. This kind of confidence is not about thinking you are perfect. It is about knowing that you can figure things out, learn new things, and pick yourself up if you stumble. It gives you the courage to say yes to new opportunities and not let fear hold you back.

Everybody faces failure and disappointment. But if you have inner strength, these moments do not break you. Instead, they teach you important lessons. Maybe you miss out on a job, or a friendship ends, or a plan falls apart. You might feel sad or upset at first, but you do not stay down for long. Reflect on what happened, learn from it, and keep moving forward. In time, you realize that every challenge made you stronger than you were before.

Another remarkable aspect of inner strength is its positive impact on your relationships. When you feel good about yourself, you do not have to pretend or hide your feelings. You can be honest and open with others. You can listen and support your loved ones, and you are not afraid to ask for help when you need it. If someone upsets you, you don't just react — you try to understand, and you work things out calmly and rationally. This makes your connections with others more real and more rewarding.

Inner strength keeps your mind positive. Even on hard days, you can find something good — a kind word, a small win, a peaceful moment. You do not let negative thoughts run the show. If you notice you are feeling down, remind yourself of your strengths or focus on what you are grateful for. This makes every day a little brighter.

You also become more independent. You do not always need others to agree with you or approve of what you do. You know what matters to you, and you can stand up for yourself in a kind and transparent manner. It becomes easier to say "no" when you need to, and you do not get pushed into things you do not want.

Most of all, inner strength helps you grow as a person. You become braver, wiser, and more comfortable with who you are. Every time you face a challenge and persevere, you become even stronger within. Life feels more hopeful and more enjoyable because you know you have what it takes — no matter what comes your way.

CHAPTER 2

Overcoming Self-Doubt

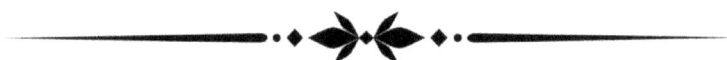

———··◆·◀◆·◆··———

Self-doubt can make even the strongest person feel unsure. It whispers that you are not good enough or that you might fail. The truth is, everyone faces these feelings at some point, but you don't have to let them hold you back. This chapter will help you understand the origins of self-doubt and offer you practical ways to manage it. You will learn how to build trust in yourself, recognize your actual abilities, and take small steps toward developing confidence. With each new skill, you will discover that you are much stronger than your doubts.

What Is Self-Doubt and Where Does It Come From?

Self-doubt is the feeling you get when you question your abilities, decisions, or worth. It is that little voice in your head that asks, "What if I mess up?" or "What if I am not good enough?" Sometimes, self-doubt is quiet and only appears occasionally. At other times, it can feel loud and constant, making it difficult to move forward or enjoy your life.

Self-doubt can manifest in various ways. Perhaps you are hesitant to try something new because you fear failure. You may not speak up in class or at work because you are worried people will laugh or disagree. You might even compare yourself to others and feel like you do not measure up. Self-doubt can make you avoid challenges, hide your true self, or settle for less than you deserve.

But where does this feeling come from? Self-doubt usually does not start overnight. Often, it begins in childhood or during times when you felt judged or not accepted. If you were frequently criticized, ignored, or told you were not good enough, these words can stick in your mind. Even small comments from teachers, parents, or friends can plant seeds of doubt that grow over time.

Life experiences can also add to self-doubt. If you have failed at something important to you, you might remember that feeling for a long time. One bad grade, a lost job, or a broken friendship can make you question yourself. Even watching others succeed while you struggle can evoke self-doubt, prompting you to wonder why things seem more complicated for you.

Another reason self-doubt is common is that our minds try to protect us from pain or embarrassment. That little voice of doubt might be trying to keep you safe from making a mistake or from feeling hurt. While this is natural, it can also keep you from growing and learning. If you always listen to your doubts, you might never find out how much you can do.

Social media and today's fast-paced world can also add to self-doubt. When you see pictures of perfect lives online or hear about other people's significant achievements, it is easy to feel left out or not good enough. You might forget that everyone has struggles and that what you see online is often not the whole story.

It is essential to recognize that having self-doubt does not mean you are weak or flawed. It means you are human. Everyone feels unsure at times, even those who appear confident on the outside. The good news is that self-doubt can be managed and even turned into a strength. By recognizing where your doubt originates, you can begin to challenge it and cultivate a more kind and realistic view of yourself.

Understanding self-doubt is the first step in overcoming it. Once you know how it works and why it appears, you can begin making choices that help build your confidence. With time and practice, you will learn that you have the power to quiet your doubts and trust yourself more with each new day.

The Impact of Self-Doubt on Daily Life

Self-doubt does not just reside in your mind; it often infiltrates almost every aspect of your day. When you feel unsure about yourself, it can change the way you act, the choices you make, and even how you think about your future. Many people do not realize the extent to which self-doubt influences their daily life until they pause to reflect on it.

One of the first places self-doubt shows up is in decision-making. When you question your judgment, even small choices can feel stressful. You might spend a long time picking out clothes in the morning or worry about whether you said the right thing to someone the day before. Big decisions — like applying for a new job, starting a project, or sharing your opinion — can feel almost impossible. Self-doubt often makes you second-guess yourself or put things off because you are afraid of making a mistake.

Self-doubt also makes it harder to try new things. If you are constantly worried about failing, you may avoid activities that could help you grow and develop. You might stay away from sports, classes, or social events because you think you will not be good enough or will embarrass yourself. Over time, this can limit your experiences and keep you stuck in the same place.

When you experience a lot of self-doubt, your confidence begins to wane. This can affect your work or school life. You might not speak up in meetings or class, even when you have good ideas. You may not pursue new opportunities because you do not believe you deserve them or are capable of handling them. You might work extra hard, trying to prove yourself, but still feel like nothing you do is ever enough. This can lead to stress, anxiety, and even burnout.

Self-doubt can also hurt your relationships with others. When you do not feel good about yourself, you may find it hard to trust people or believe that they like you. You might read too much into small comments or worry that friends or family are judging you. Sometimes, self-doubt makes you keep your real feelings or needs a secret, because you are afraid of being rejected or misunderstood. This can make you feel lonely, even when you're surrounded by people.

Another way self-doubt affects daily life is by feeding negative self-talk. You might catch yourself thinking, "I always mess up," or "I am not as smart as everyone else." These thoughts can become a habit, running through your mind without you even noticing. Over time, they can lower your mood, drain your energy, and diminish your enthusiasm for your goals.

Self-doubt can even affect your health. When you worry a lot or feel bad about yourself, your body feels it too. You may experience trouble sleeping, headaches, or feel tired all the time. Some people struggle to eat well or exercise because they lack motivation or doubt their ability to succeed.

The truth is, self-doubt can touch almost every part of your life. It can hold you back from growing, make you feel stuck, and keep you from enjoying the good things that come your way. But once you recognize how much it affects you, you can start to make changes. Each time you notice self-doubt, you have a chance to challenge it and choose a kinder thought or a braver action.

Learning to notice and manage self-doubt takes practice, but it can change your life in big and small ways. As you build more trust in yourself, you will find it easier to make decisions, try new things, and enjoy your day-to-day life. Remember, everyone struggles with doubt sometimes, but you do not have to let it run your life. You can learn to believe in yourself, step by step, and discover just how much you can do.

Strategies to Challenge Negative Self-Talk

Negative self-talk occurs when you repeatedly tell yourself things like "I'm not good enough" or "I always mess up." These thoughts can feel true, but most of the time, they are not. They are just habits your mind has learned over time. The good news is, you can change these habits and start being kinder to yourself. Here are some simple ways to challenge negative self-talk:

First, pay attention to what you are saying in your head. Sometimes, you might not even notice these thoughts because they occur so quickly. Try to catch yourself when you think, "I can't do this," or "I'm not as smart as others." You do not need to stop the thought right away—notice it. This is the first step in making the change.

Next, ask yourself if the thought is actual. Imagine a friend came to you with the same worry. What would you say to them? Would you agree with their negative thought, or would you remind them of their good qualities? Often, you will find that your mind is being too hard on you. Treat yourself with the same kindness you would offer a friend.

You can also look for objective evidence. For example, if you think, "I never do anything right," stop and think of times when you did something well. Perhaps you helped someone, completed a challenging task, or made someone smile. Remind yourself that everyone makes mistakes sometimes, but that does not mean you always fail.

Another helpful trick is to replace a negative thought with a more positive or balanced one. Instead of saying, "I always mess up," try, "Sometimes I make mistakes, but I can learn and improve." Instead of "I'm not good enough," try "I am still learning, and that's okay." It may feel strange at first, but the more you practice, the more natural it will feel.

Writing down your thoughts can also be helpful. If you have a lot of negative self-talk, try writing the thoughts in a notebook and then writing a kinder response next to each one. For example, if you write, "I'm so bad at talking to people," you could answer, "I am trying, and every conversation helps me get better." Seeing your thoughts on paper makes it easier to identify those that are too harsh or unfair.

Finally, practice being patient with yourself. Changing the way you think takes time and effort. If you catch yourself slipping back into old habits, do not get upset. Just notice it and gently bring your mind back to a kinder thought. Remember, everyone talks down to themselves sometimes, but you don't have to listen to or believe everything you think.

Each time you challenge a negative thought, you are teaching your mind a new way to see yourself. Bit by bit, you will start to notice more good things about yourself and feel more confident in what you can do.

Building Confidence through Action

Confidence is not something that magically appears. It is something you build, little by little, by taking real steps in your everyday life. Many people wait to feel confident before they start something new, but the secret is this: confidence comes *after* you take action, not before.

Think about a time you learned to ride a bike or speak in front of a group. At first, you probably felt nervous, maybe even scared. But with each try, you became a bit braver. The first time was shaky. The second time, you might have wobbled but did not fall. By the third or fourth time, it started to feel possible. That is how confidence grows—by doing, by practicing, and by not giving up.

You do not need to start with a giant leap. Small actions matter just as much, maybe even more. If speaking up in meetings feels scary, you can start by sharing your ideas with one friendly coworker or sending your thoughts in a message. If you want to get fit, you do not need to run a marathon. Just put on your shoes and go for a short walk. These small actions might seem simple, but each one is a building block for your self-belief.

Sometimes, the hardest part is just beginning. You might worry that you will make a mistake or that others will judge you. However, the truth is that nobody gets it perfect the first time. Every expert started as a beginner. The more you act, the more you realize that mistakes are part of the process, not a reason to quit, but a lesson to learn from.

Setting small, clear goals can make action feel less overwhelming. Choose goals that you can reach so that you can feel proud of yourself often. For example, if you want to become a better public speaker, your first goal might be to introduce yourself to someone new. Celebrate that step! Next, share one idea in a group. With each new action, you will notice that your courage grows. Celebrate every step forward, no matter how small.

Sometimes you will stumble. That is normal. Instead of telling yourself, "I failed," try saying, "I tried, and now I know more than before." Mistakes do not mean you cannot do it. They tell you that you are learning, growing, and giving yourself a chance to get better. Confidence is built through trying, not by getting everything right.

It also helps to have people around you who cheer you on. Share your goal with a friend or family member and let them offer encouragement. Sometimes, hearing someone say, "You can do it!" is the push you need to take action.

Over time, all these small steps add up. You will notice that things that once made you nervous start to feel normal. You will find yourself taking on bigger challenges, not because you are never scared, but because you have learned that you can handle it.

Building confidence is an adventure, not a race. Every action you take, no matter how small, is a victory. With each step, you are teaching yourself that you are capable, brave, and ready for more. Before you know it, you will look back and see how far you have come—all because you decided to take that very first step.

Self-Compassion as a Tool for Healing

Being kind to yourself is one of the most important ways to heal from self-doubt and grow stronger inside. Self-compassion means treating yourself with the same care and understanding you would offer a good friend. It is about letting go of harsh self-judgment and choosing patience, even when you make mistakes.

When something goes wrong, it's easy to blame yourself or think you're not good enough. You might say things in your mind that you would never say to someone else. This can hurt even more than the original mistake. Self-compassion is the opposite. It is stopping for a moment, taking a breath, and reminding yourself that everyone has hard days and everyone makes errors sometimes. You are not alone.

Showing compassion to yourself does not mean ignoring your problems or never trying to improve. It means you accept that being human means having ups and downs. When you mess up, instead of saying, "I am a failure," try saying, "I am learning, and it is okay to make mistakes." This gentle attitude helps you recover from setbacks and builds a strong foundation for growth.

You can practice self-compassion in simple ways every day. Start by noticing your thoughts. If you catch yourself being too hard on yourself, pause and ask, "Would I say this to a friend?" If the answer is no, try to rephrase your words in a more caring manner. You might say, "This is hard, but I am doing my best," or "I am proud of myself for trying."

Taking care of your body is another form of self-compassion. Get enough sleep, eat healthy foods, and take breaks when needed. Listen to what your body and mind are telling you. If you need help, reach out to someone you trust.

It also helps to remember that you are not alone in your struggles. Everyone faces challenges, and everyone feels insecure sometimes. When you recognize this, it becomes easier to forgive yourself and move forward.

Over time, self-compassion can help heal old wounds and bring new confidence. You become less afraid of making mistakes because you know you can handle them kindly. You start to see your worth, not because you are perfect, but because you are human. Each small act of kindness to yourself adds up, helping you feel calmer, stronger, and more hopeful about the future.

Self-compassion is a powerful tool. It turns self-doubt into self-care and helps you build the inner strength you need to face whatever comes next.

Real-Life Stories of Overcoming Self-Doubt

Sometimes, the best way to understand self-doubt is to see how real people have faced it and come out stronger. Here are a few short stories of everyday people who learned to move past their doubts and believe in themselves.

Aisha always wanted to learn how to paint, but she was afraid her art would not be good enough. Every time she picked up a brush, she worried others would laugh at her work. One day, a friend invited her to a local art class. At first, Aisha felt shy and almost did not go. But she decided to give it a try. With each painting, she learned that the joy was in creating, not in being perfect. Slowly, her confidence grew. Now, Aisha paints every week and even shares her artwork online, inspiring others to try something new.

Another story is about Salman, who dreamed of speaking in front of a crowd but was terrified of making mistakes. He used to think, "I am not a good speaker. People will think I am boring." Instead of avoiding public speaking, Salman decided to practice in small ways. He joined a local group where members supported each other. The first time, his hands shook and he forgot some words. But the group cheered him on. Each time he spoke, his self-doubt became a little quieter. Today, Salman gives talks at community events, and he takes pride in the progress he has made.

Fatima faced self-doubt when she applied for a new job. She kept thinking, "I am not as smart as the other candidates. I probably will not get the job." But she reminded herself of her hard work and the skills she had built. She prepared carefully and went to the interview. To her surprise, she got the job! Fatima realized that everyone has doubts, but taking a chance can lead to incredible opportunities.

These stories demonstrate that self-doubt is a natural part of life, but it doesn't have to hold you back. Each person started small, tried new things, and accepted their mistakes along the way. The most crucial step was believing that growth is possible. By taking action, asking for help, and being kind to themselves, they each discovered strengths they had not known they possessed.

Your story can be just as powerful. The first step is to notice your self-doubt and then choose to move forward anyway. With practice and patience, you can write your own story of overcoming self-doubt—one brave step at a time.

CHAPTER 3

Developing a Growth Mindset

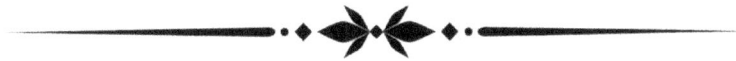

A growth mindset means believing you can learn and improve through effort and practice. It is the idea that your abilities are not fixed—they can grow as you face new challenges and learn from your mistakes. In this chapter, you will discover how your thoughts shape your confidence and success. With a growth mindset, setbacks become opportunities for learning and growth, rather than reasons to quit. You will learn simple ways to change your thinking and view every challenge as an opportunity to become better, stronger, and wiser. This new mindset can help you achieve your goals and enjoy the learning process along the way.

Growth Mindset vs. Fixed Mindset

There are two primary ways people perceive their abilities. One approach is known as a growth mindset. This means you believe you can get better at something with practice, effort, and learning. You know that you might not be good at something right away, but you can improve if you keep trying. With a growth mindset, you do not let mistakes stop you. Instead, you see them as chances to learn and grow.

The other way of thinking is called a fixed mindset. People with a fixed mindset believe their talents, intelligence, or skills are fixed—they are either what they are or they are not. If they find something challenging, they might give up easily or avoid trying because they think, "I am just not good at this." They may feel embarrassed by mistakes or see failure as proof that they cannot succeed.

These two mindsets can make a big difference in your life. For example, if you have a growth mindset and you do not do well on a test, you might say, "I can study more and do better next time." But with a fixed mindset, you might think, "I am not smart enough for this," and stop trying. The first way helps you keep moving forward, while the second way can hold you back.

It is essential to recognize the mindset you use most frequently. You might find that in some areas, like sports or art, you believe you can improve, but in others, like math or public speaking, you feel stuck. The good news is that you can choose to cultivate a growth mindset in any part of your life. It starts with believing that your brain can grow and change, just like a muscle gets stronger when you exercise it.

When you adopt a growth mindset, challenges become exciting rather than scary. You become braver, more willing to try new things, and more able to enjoy learning. Over time, you start to see that effort does make a difference, and you feel more confident facing whatever comes your way.

Growth Mindset	Fixed Mindset
Believes skills can improve with effort	Thinks skills and talents are unchangeable
Sees mistakes as chances to learn	Sees mistakes as proof of failure
Tries new things, even if they are hard	Avoids challenges that seem difficult
Says "I can get better if I practice"	Says "I am just not good at this"
Keeps going after setbacks	Gives up easily when things go wrong
Enjoys learning and growing	Wants to look smart or avoid embarrassment
Accepts feedback as helpful advice	Sees feedback as criticism or a personal attack

Recognizing Your Own Mindset

Recognizing your mindset is the first big step in building a more positive and successful life. Everyone has thoughts that come from both a growth mindset and a fixed mindset, but most people are not fully aware of which one guides them more often. Paying close attention to your thoughts, words, and reactions can help you find out which mindset is shaping your choices and actions.

Start by noticing how you respond to challenges or difficult situations. Imagine learning something new, such as riding a bike, starting a new job, or studying a challenging subject at school. When you make a mistake or feel stuck, what goes through your mind? If you think, "I am just not good at this," "I will never get it," or "Maybe this just is not for me," these are signs of a fixed mindset. These thoughts make it easy to give up or avoid trying altogether.

On the other hand, if you hear yourself saying, "This is hard, but I can get better with practice," "Mistakes help me learn," or "I am going to try again and see if I improve," these are growth mindset thoughts. They show you are willing to put in effort and believe you can improve over time, even if things are not easy right away.

A good way to recognize your mindset is to pay attention to your "self-talk"—the silent conversations you have in your head every day. When you face something challenging, do you encourage yourself or put yourself down? For example, do you say, "I always mess up," or do you say, "Everyone makes mistakes, and I can learn from this one"? The words you use, even if only in your mind, have a significant effect on how you feel and what you do next.

You can also look for patterns in how you react to feedback or criticism. People with a fixed mindset often feel upset, embarrassed, or even angry when they hear something negative about their work. They might think, "I am just not smart enough," or "They do not understand me." People with a growth mindset, however, view feedback as a valuable tool for growth. They think, "This can help me get better," or, "What can I learn from this?" By being open to feedback, you are showing that you believe in your ability to grow.

Notice your reactions when you see others succeed. Do you feel jealous or discouraged, thinking you will never be as good? That is a sign of a fixed mindset. If you feel inspired by others' success and start thinking, "If they can do it, maybe I can too," that is a growth mindset at work.

Another way to recognize your mindset is to notice how you approach new opportunities. Do you avoid trying new things because you are afraid you will fail, or do you give them a shot, even if you are nervous? If you catch yourself thinking, "I might as well not try," that is a fixed mindset. But if you try anyway to learn and see what happens, you are using a growth mindset.

It helps to write down your thoughts and feelings, especially when you feel stuck, frustrated, or challenged. Keep a small notebook or use your phone to jot down your reactions. Over time, you will notice which kind of mindset emerges most frequently.

Recognizing your mindset is powerful because it gives you the chance to change it. If you notice fixed-mindset thoughts, you do not have to believe them or let them control you. You can choose to talk back to those thoughts with something more hopeful and faithful. For example, instead of thinking, "I can't do this," try saying, "I can't do this yet, but I can learn."

Bit by bit, as you become more aware of your thoughts and adopt a growth mindset more frequently, you will notice changes in your confidence, your willingness to try new things, and your enjoyment of learning. It all begins with paying attention to your mind and being honest about what you find.

Steps to Shift Your Perspective

Shifting your perspective from a fixed mindset to a growth mindset is like opening a window and letting fresh air into a stuffy room. It takes practice, but each small step brings more light and hope into your life. Here are some simple, practical steps you can use to start changing the way you think:

The first step is to listen to your thoughts. When you face a challenge or make a mistake, pause and notice what you say to yourself. Do you think things like "I'll never get this right" or "I'm just not good at this"? If so, that is your fixed mindset talking. Becoming aware of these thoughts is important because you cannot change what you do not notice.

Once you have noticed a negative or fixed mindset thought, try to question it. Ask yourself, "Is this really true, or am I just feeling discouraged right now?" Most of the time, the answer is that you are being too hard on yourself. Remind yourself that nobody is perfect and that learning is a process that takes time to develop.

A powerful way to shift your thinking is to add the word "yet" to your thoughts. For example, change "I can't do this" to "I can't do this yet." That one small word can open the door to new possibilities and help your brain believe that improvement is possible with effort and time.

Focus on the process, not just the result. When you prioritize winning, being perfect, or reaching the end goal, it is easy to feel discouraged by setbacks. Instead, try to notice and celebrate your effort, progress, and what you're learning along the way. Each small step forward counts, even if you have not reached your big goal yet.

Another critical step is to turn mistakes into lessons. Instead of seeing failure as the end, ask yourself, "What can I learn from this?" Every mistake is an opportunity to learn more, grow stronger, and try a new approach next time. The more you practice this, the less afraid you become of trying new things.

Surround yourself with people who encourage growth. Spend time with friends, teachers, or family members who support you and believe in learning and trying new things. Their positive attitude can help you see challenges in a new light and keep you motivated when things get tough.

Try to use kind and supportive language with yourself. If you catch yourself thinking something negative, gently change it to something more hopeful. For example, "This is too hard" can become, "This is hard, but I can try and improve." Treat yourself the way you would treat a friend who is struggling.

Practice gratitude for your efforts, even when things do not work out right away. Thank yourself for showing up, for trying, and for not giving up. Gratitude helps you see how far you have come, and it keeps your mind open to learning more.

Be patient with yourself. Changing your perspective will not happen overnight. Some days, you may slip back into old habits, and that's okay. The important thing is to keep going, keep learning, and keep believing that you can grow.

Each of these steps, practiced over time, will help shift your perspective and build a proper growth mindset. The more you do it, the more natural it will become—and the more you will discover about what you are truly capable of.

Learning from Failure and Mistakes

No one likes to fail, but the truth is that mistakes are a regular part of life. Everyone, even the most successful people, fails at something along the way. What matters most is not the mistake itself, but what you do after it happens. If you view your failures as learning opportunities, you can grow stronger and wiser with each one.

When you make a mistake, it's easy to feel disappointed, embarrassed, or even angry with yourself. These feelings are normal. But instead of letting them hold you back, you can choose to see the mistake as a lesson. Ask yourself, "What can I learn from this?" You may discover a new way to solve a problem or notice something you can do differently next time. Each mistake provides you with valuable information that can help you improve.

Sometimes, people worry that making mistakes means they are not good enough. However, everyone makes mistakes, regardless of how smart or talented they are. Some of the world's greatest inventors, artists, and athletes failed many times before reaching their goals. What made them successful was not that they never failed, but that they kept going and continued to learn from their mistakes.

Try to be gentle with yourself when things do not work out. Remind yourself that it's okay to make mistakes and that you're still growing. If you make a mistake, it doesn't mean you're a failure—it means you're human. Give yourself credit for trying, and remember that each effort brings you closer to your goal.

If you are stuck after a failure, talk to someone you trust. A friend, teacher, or family member can help you see the situation from a different perspective. Sometimes, just talking about it makes it easier to spot the lesson hidden inside the mistake.

It also helps to remember your past successes. Think about other times you made mistakes and learned from them. How did you overcome those moments? What did you do differently afterward? Use those experiences as proof that you can handle challenges and continue to grow.

Celebrate your effort, even if the result was not perfect. Trying new things and taking risks is a brave choice. Each time you face a challenge, you build resilience and courage—even when you do not win or get everything right.

Learning from failure is a powerful skill. Instead of letting mistakes make you give up, use them as stepping stones toward success. Each lesson you know brings you one step closer to your dreams. With this mindset, you will see that mistakes are not the end—they are the beginning of something better.

Tools for Sustaining a Growth Mindset

Building a growth mindset is an excellent start, but maintaining that mindset requires a little effort each day. When you use simple tools and make a few healthy habits part of your routine, you can keep your belief in learning and growing steady, even during tough times.

One of the most potent tools is positive self-talk. The way you speak to yourself, even in your mind, can lift you or hold you back. Start your day with encouraging words, such as "I can improve with practice," or "Each mistake helps me grow." If you catch yourself thinking, "I can't do this," gently add the word "yet": "I can't do this yet, but I am learning." Over time, these new messages will replace the old, negative ones, making it easier to stay motivated.

Goal setting is another essential tool. Instead of setting one huge goal that feels overwhelming, break your big dream into smaller, straightforward steps. Each time you reach a small goal, take a moment to celebrate your effort. This could mean telling yourself, "I did it!" or treating yourself to something you enjoy. These small wins add up, making progress easier to see and feel. When you celebrate effort instead of just the result, you train your mind to value learning and persistence.

Keeping a journal is a simple yet highly beneficial habit. You can write about your thoughts after a tough day, or make a list of things you learned from a mistake. Journaling helps you spot patterns in your thinking and see your growth over time. Try writing down three things you did well each week, and notice how your mindset shifts toward a more positive outlook.

Being open to feedback is a powerful way to maintain a strong growth mindset. Instead of feeling hurt by advice or criticism, use it as a chance to improve. Ask, "What can I learn from this?" and "How can I use this feedback next time?" Feedback from teachers, mentors, or friends is like a map that helps you find better ways to reach your goals.

Learning from others is another great habit. Look for people who inspire you—maybe a coach, a classmate, or someone in your family. Watch how they handle setbacks and keep working toward their dreams. Their stories can show you that hard work pays off and that everyone faces challenges. Use their example to remind yourself that effort matters more than perfection.

Reflection is another essential tool. Set aside a little time each week to reflect on what went well and what challenges you faced. Ask yourself questions like, "What did I learn?" and "How can I use this lesson next time?" Reflection helps you focus on growth rather than just results, and it shows you that progress is possible even when things are challenging.

Surrounding yourself with people who believe in growth can make a big difference. Find friends or family who encourage you to keep trying and celebrate your progress. A positive group can help you stay strong, especially on days when you feel stuck.

Remember to be patient and kind with yourself. Growth takes time, and setbacks are an inevitable part of the learning process. If you have a tough day, remind yourself that you can always try again tomorrow. Every bit of effort you put in helps you get stronger, wiser, and more confident.

With these tools and habits, you can cultivate and maintain a growth mindset. Each day presents a new opportunity to learn, grow, and savor the journey of becoming your best self.

CHAPTER 4

Embracing Change

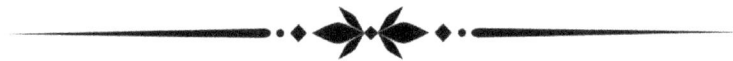

———··◆◆··———

Change is a natural part of life. Sometimes it arrives when you expect it, but often it shows up when you least expect it. Change can be both exciting and intimidating, as it can also feel scary, confusing, or overwhelming. You may need to start a new school, relocate to a new place, switch jobs, or adapt to changes in your family or health. Even positive changes can make you feel nervous or unsure.

This chapter explores why change is so challenging and how you can learn to accept it instead of fighting against it. You will find simple ideas and real-life tips to help you handle changes, big and small, with more courage and calm. By learning how to face change with an open mind, you can find new opportunities, grow stronger, and move forward with confidence—even when life takes you in a new direction.

Why Change Is Difficult

Change can be hard for almost everyone, even if the change is something you wanted. One big reason is that people like to feel safe and comfortable. When life is predictable, you know what to expect and how to handle things. Change, on the other hand, brings something new and unknown. It can make you feel like you're not in control, and that feeling can be unsettling.

Another reason change is difficult is that it often means leaving something behind. This could be a routine, a place, a friendship, or even just the way things used to be. Even if the old way was not perfect, it was familiar. Letting go can bring up feelings of sadness, worry, or even anger.

Change can also make you doubt yourself. You might wonder, "Can I handle this?" or "What if things do not work out?" These thoughts can make you want to stay where you are, even if you are not happy or growing.

Sometimes, people are afraid of making mistakes when things change. You might worry about failing or looking silly in front of others. This fear can keep you from trying new things or from moving forward when change is needed.

It is also natural for your mind to focus on what might go wrong instead of what could go right. This is referred to as "negative thinking," and it is a common phenomenon during times of change. Your brain is simply trying to protect you from getting hurt, but it can also make change seem bigger and scarier than it is.

Finally, change can be hard because it takes energy and effort. You have to learn new things, build new habits, and sometimes start from scratch. This process can be tiring, especially when multiple changes co-occur.

Although change can be difficult, it also presents an opportunity to learn, grow, and discover new aspects of yourself. Understanding why change feels so hard is the first step in learning how to handle it with more strength and confidence.

Emotional Reactions to Change

When life changes, your emotions often change too. It is normal to experience a range of emotions during times of change. You might feel excited about what is coming, but you could also feel scared, sad, or even angry. Sometimes you may feel all of these at once, and that is okay.

People often feel worried or anxious when they are uncertain about what will happen next. You might wonder, "Will I be able to handle this?" or "What if things go wrong?" These thoughts can cause your heart to race or your stomach to feel tight. Feeling nervous about the unknown is a widespread experience.

Sadness can show up when you have to let go of something familiar, like an old routine, a friendship, or a place you love. Even if you know the change is good, you might still miss how things used to be. This sadness is a natural part of the process.

Sometimes, you might feel frustrated or angry, especially if you did not choose the change or if it feels unfair. It is normal to wish things could stay the same. You may even feel upset with yourself or others for not being able to control the situation.

Remember, all of these feelings are normal. Everyone reacts differently to change. It is essential to permit yourself to feel your emotions without judgment. Talking about your feelings with someone you trust can help, and so can writing them down. Over time, as you adjust, your emotions will settle, and you will find new ways to feel comfortable and confident again.

Techniques to Become More Adaptable

Being adaptable means you can adjust to new situations, even when they are unexpected or challenging. Adaptability helps you stay calm, think clearly, and find solutions, regardless of the changes life brings. Here are some simple techniques to help you become more adaptable:

Start by practicing an open mind. When something changes, try not to say, "This will never work," right away. Instead, ask yourself, "What can I learn from this?" or "Is there a new way to solve this problem?" Even if you feel unsure, reminding yourself to be curious can make change less scary.

Stay flexible with your plans. It is good to have goals, but sometimes things do not go as expected. If your plan changes, try to see it as a new adventure instead of a disaster. Look for the good in the situation, even if it is something small. Flexibility helps you move forward without feeling stuck.

Build new skills whenever you can. When you learn something new — like cooking a meal, fixing a small problem, or even using new technology — you show yourself that you can handle change. Every new skill, no matter how small, makes you more confident and adaptable.

Focus on what you can control, and try not to stress about what you cannot. When something changes, write down the things you can do to help yourself adjust. This might mean asking for advice, making a new plan, or taking a small step each day. Let go of things you cannot change, like other people's choices or unexpected events.

Practice staying calm when things go wrong. Take slow, deep breaths, count to ten, or step outside for some fresh air. When you are relaxed, you can think more clearly and make better choices. It is okay to feel upset, but calming your body can help you handle the change with more strength.

Ask for help if you need it. Being adaptable does not mean you have to do everything alone. Friends, family, and teachers can offer new ideas and support. Sometimes, simply discussing a problem can help you view it in a new and more insightful light.

Remind yourself of past changes you have handled well. Think about a time when you were nervous about something new, but it turned out okay. Remembering your strengths gives you the courage to face new changes.

Be kind to yourself. Change is challenging for everyone, and it takes time to adjust to new things. Celebrate your progress, even if it's small, and trust that you will become more adaptable with every new experience.

With these techniques, you can build adaptability and feel ready for whatever changes come your way.

How to Use Change for Growth

Change is something that everyone faces, sometimes when they least expect it. While it can often feel scary or uncomfortable, change is also a powerful force for personal growth. When you learn how to use change to your advantage, you can discover new strengths, build confidence, and find opportunities you never imagined.

One of the first steps in embracing change for growth is to recognize that change is an inherent part of life. Everything around us changes—seasons shift, people grow older, new technology arrives, and routines adjust. When you accept this fact, you begin to see change as something natural, rather than something to fear. This acceptance helps you relax and be more open to new experiences.

Whenever change happens, it helps to pause and notice your feelings. You might feel sad, nervous, excited, or confused. All of these emotions are valid. Take time to listen to yourself. Ask, "What am I feeling right now? Why do I feel this way?" Sometimes, naming your emotions makes them feel less overwhelming. Once you understand your feelings, you can make choices that help you move forward instead of feeling stuck.

The next step is to look for the lessons inside the change. Every change—good or bad—teaches you something new. For example, if you move to a new city, you might learn how to make new friends, explore a new place, and become more independent. If you lose a job, you may discover new skills or passions that lead you in a better direction. Even complex changes show you what you are capable of handling and can help you grow stronger.

It is also essential to ask yourself, "How can I make the most of this change?" The change may not be something you chose, but you can still choose your attitude and the actions that follow. For instance, if your daily routine changes, look for small ways to take care of yourself, like starting a new hobby, joining a club, or spending more time with loved ones. These small choices help you feel more in control and open the door to positive growth.

Trying new things is a powerful way to use change for growth. When life shifts, it is the perfect time to step out of your comfort zone. Sign up for a class, learn a new skill, or explore a different place. Even if it feels uncomfortable at first, you will gain confidence as you try new things and succeed in unexpected ways.

Another essential aspect of growing through change is maintaining a positive outlook. This does not mean ignoring problems or pretending everything is perfect. Instead, it means looking for something good, even in tough times. Ask yourself, "What can I be grateful for right now?" or "Is there a silver lining in this situation?" Focusing on gratitude and hope helps you maintain your spirits and see new possibilities, even when life feels challenging.

Building a support system can make a significant difference during times of change. Talk to friends, family, teachers, or anyone you trust. Share your feelings, ask for advice, and listen to their stories about how they handled changes in their own lives. Sometimes, just knowing you are not alone can help you feel stronger and more confident about facing what's ahead.

Change can also teach you about your resilience. Each time you face something new and get through it, you build inner strength. You learn to trust yourself, knowing that you can handle more than you thought possible. Over time, you begin to welcome change as an opportunity to grow and become your best self.

That growth does not happen all at once. Be patient with yourself as you adjust to this new situation. There will be ups and downs, but each step forward counts. Celebrate your progress, no matter how small, and trust that every change brings a new opportunity to learn and become stronger.

Accepting change, looking for the lessons, staying positive, and taking brave steps forward, you can use every change as a tool for growth. Life will always be in a state of constant change, but with the right mindset, you can continue to grow right along with it.

Stories of Transformational Change

Sometimes, the best way to understand how change can help us grow is to hear real-life stories from people who faced significant changes and emerged stronger on the other side. These stories demonstrate that while change can be intimidating, it can also open doors you never thought possible.

One story is about Sara, who had lived in the same small town her whole life. When her parents got new jobs in a different city, Sara had to leave her friends and everything she knew. At first, she felt lost and worried she would never feel at home again. But with time, Sara began exploring her new neighborhood, joining a local art club, and making friends at her new school. She discovered a love for painting and even won a local art contest. Looking back, Sara realized that the move taught her she could handle new situations and find happiness wherever she went.

Another story is about Ahmed, who lost his job after the company he worked for closed down. Ahmed felt discouraged and scared about the future. But instead of giving up, he decided to use this unexpected change as a chance to learn something new. He began taking online courses in graphic design, a subject he had always enjoyed but had never pursued seriously. With hard work and practice, Ahmed became skilled enough to start his own small business. Not only did he find a new career he loved, but he also gained confidence in his ability to handle setbacks and try new things.

Fatima's story is about personal change. She used to be very shy and was afraid to speak up in groups. When her best friend moved away, Fatima felt even more alone. She decided to join a local community group, despite feeling nervous. At first, it was hard for her to talk to new people, but the more she participated, the more comfortable she became. Over time, Fatima made close friends and even started leading small group meetings. The experience helped her realize that change could reveal strengths she had never known she possessed.

Each of these stories demonstrates that even though change is challenging, it can lead to remarkable growth. Sara, Ahmed, and Fatima all faced moments when they felt afraid or uncertain. However, by taking small steps forward, asking for help when needed, and giving themselves time to adjust, they each found new confidence and happiness.

Your story can be just as powerful. When you face a significant change, remember that you don't have to do it all at once. Take it one day at a time. Look for small ways to learn, connect, and grow. Change is not just something to survive; it is something that can help you become the best version of yourself.

CHAPTER 5

Setting Goals

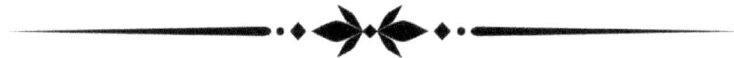

Everyone dreams of doing something special, but dreams become real when you turn them into goals. Setting goals gives your life direction, purpose, and energy. Goals are like a map—they show you where you want to go and help you figure out the best way to get there. Whether your goal is big or small, having a clear target gives you something to work toward, making every step feel meaningful.

This chapter will explain why setting goals is essential, how to select the right goals for yourself, and how to stay motivated even when the path becomes challenging. You will learn simple, practical ways to turn your wishes into plans and your plans into action. By the end of this chapter, you will see that reaching your goals is not about luck—it is about taking clear steps, one after another, and believing in your power to succeed.

The Science behind Goal Setting

Setting goals is not just about writing down what you want—it is backed by science. Research indicates that individuals who set clear goals are significantly more likely to achieve their desired outcomes in life. This is because having a goal gives your mind something to focus on. It helps you pay attention to what matters and block out distractions.

When you set a goal, your brain begins searching for ways to achieve it. You become more aware of opportunities and solutions that can help you move forward. Even small goals can give you a sense of purpose and direction each day.

Scientists have also found that setting specific, realistic goals helps you stay motivated. When you break a big goal into smaller steps, each small win gives your brain a burst of positive energy. This makes you feel proud of your progress and keeps you excited to keep going.

Writing down your goals is another powerful tool. Research indicates that individuals who write down their goals are more likely to achieve them. It helps you remember what you want, track your progress, and stay committed—especially when things get hard.

Goals also help you bounce back from setbacks. When you know what you are working toward, it is easier to stay focused and find new ways to persevere, even when facing challenges. This is why athletes, students, and successful individuals in all fields utilize goal setting as a key component of their growth.

Setting goals gives your life structure and helps you turn dreams into action. The science is precise: having goals makes you more confident, motivated, and ready to reach your full potential.

How to Set SMART Goals

Setting goals is powerful, but not all goals are equally effective. To make your goals truly effective, try using the SMART method. SMART goals are clear and well-planned, so you know exactly what you want and how to get there. Here's what SMART stands for:

Specific

Your goal should be clear and focused. Instead of saying, "I want to get healthier," you could say, "I want to walk 30 minutes every day." The more detailed you are, the easier it is to know what to do next.

Measurable

A good goal lets you track your progress. Ask yourself, "How will I know when I reach my goal?" For example, "I will drink eight glasses of water every day" is something that can be measured. This helps you see how far you have come.

Achievable

Pick a goal that you can realistically reach. It should challenge you, but not be impossible. For example, if you want to save money, set a goal that fits your budget, like "I will save 500 rupees each month." Achievable goals keep you motivated because you know you can succeed.

Relevant

Ensure your goal aligns with your values and meets your needs. If a goal is essential to you, you are more likely to stick with it. Think about why the goal matters in your life right now.

Time-bound

Set a deadline for your goal. A clear time limit keeps you focused and helps you avoid procrastination. For example, "I will finish reading my new book in two weeks." A deadline gives you something to work toward.

When you use the SMART method, your goals become easier to follow and much more likely to succeed. Take a few minutes to write down a goal you have, and check if it's SMART. If not, adjust it using these steps. You'll find that clear, SMART goals help you stay on track and turn your wishes into tangible, achievable results.

Breaking Goals into Actionable Steps

Setting a big goal is exciting, but it can also feel overwhelming. Sometimes, just thinking about everything you need to do can make you feel stuck or even make you want to give up before you start. That is why it is crucial to break down your big goal into small, actionable steps. Each step is a piece of the puzzle that, over time, will help you reach your goal without feeling lost or discouraged.

Imagine you want to run a 5-kilometer race. That is a big goal, especially if you have never run before. If you focus solely on the finish line, it may be too distant or too challenging to reach. But if you break the goal down, it becomes much easier. Your first step might be to get a good pair of running shoes. Next, find a beginner's running plan or ask a friend to join you for support. After that, your steps could include jogging for five minutes a day, then slowly increasing your time each week. Each little action builds on the last one, and before you know it, you are much closer to running that race.

The same method applies to any goal, such as saving money, learning a new language, writing a book, or improving grades. Start by examining your primary goal and asking yourself, "What do I need to do first?" If your goal is to save a certain amount of money, your first step might be to open a savings account. Then, you can make a plan to put aside a small amount each week or month. If your goal is to write a book, your first action could be to write a simple outline, followed by writing one paragraph each day. By focusing on just one small task at a time, you make steady progress and avoid feeling overwhelmed.

It can be beneficial to create a list of all the small actions required to achieve your goal. Write these steps down in order, and put a check mark beside each one as you finish it. This does more than keep you organized — it gives you a sense of achievement every time you complete a step. Checking items off your list feels good and gives you the motivation to keep moving forward, even when the big goal still feels far away.

If you ever feel stuck, try breaking your steps down even further. For example, if writing a whole chapter for your book seems too hard, make your step even smaller: write just one paragraph or jot down some ideas for ten minutes. If saving a large amount of money feels impossible, start by putting aside a small amount each day. The important thing is to keep moving, no matter how small the action seems.

Perfection is not the goal—progress is. Some days, you will move quickly, and on other days, you may only take one small step. Both count, and both bring you closer to your dream. Celebrate your progress, no matter how small it may seem. Every action builds your confidence and reminds you that you are making progress toward success.

You may also find it helpful to share your steps with a friend, family member, or mentor who can offer encouragement and support, helping you stay accountable. When you talk about your progress with someone you trust, you are more likely to keep going, even on days when motivation is low.

Keep your list of steps visible. Please put it on your wall, in your planner, or on your phone. Looking at your steps each day is a powerful reminder that your goal is not just a dream—it is a real journey made up of many small victories.

Breaking down big goals into clear, actionable steps turns a daunting journey into a series of manageable tasks. With patience and steady effort, you will soon look back and see just how far you have come, one step at a time.

Staying Motivated and Accountable

Setting goals is an essential first step, but maintaining high energy and focus as you work toward them can be challenging. Many people feel excited at the beginning, but as days go by, they might lose motivation or forget why they started. This is normal—everyone struggles with motivation from time to time. The good news is that there are practical ways to stay motivated and hold yourself accountable, even when things get tough.

First, always remind yourself why your goal matters to you. When you have an apparent reason, you feel more connected to your goal and are more likely to persevere. Take a few moments to write down why you want to reach your goal. It may be for your health, happiness, family, or future. Read your "why" whenever you feel discouraged. Keeping your reason in mind helps you push through difficult moments and keeps your journey meaningful.

Break your big goal into smaller milestones and celebrate your wins along the way. Motivation often wanes when a goal seems too distant. By creating small checkpoints, you give yourself more chances to feel successful. For example, if your goal is to read 12 books in a year, celebrate every time you finish one. Each milestone gives you a boost of energy and reminds you that you are making progress.

Visualization is another powerful tool. Take a few minutes each day to imagine yourself reaching your goal. Picture how it will feel, what you will see, and who will be there to celebrate with you. This mental practice can make your goal feel more tangible and keep you motivated to continue working toward it.

Creating a routine or schedule also helps. Set aside specific times each week to work on your goal. Whether it's early in the morning, after dinner, or on weekends, having a regular time builds a habit and makes it easier to stay on track. Even on days when motivation is low, sticking to your routine helps you stay on track.

Accountability is crucial to achieving your goals. Find someone you trust—a friend, family member, coach, or mentor—and share your goal with them. Ask them to check in with you periodically. When you know someone else is watching your progress, you are more likely to follow through. You can also join a group or find a "goal buddy" who is working toward a similar goal. Supporting one another makes the journey easier and more enjoyable.

Keep a record of your progress. Use a journal, app, or calendar to track each step you complete. Write down what worked, what was hard, and how you felt along the way. Looking back on your progress helps you see how far you have come and encourages you to keep going, even if you have a setback.

When you face obstacles or feel like giving up, remember that setbacks are a regular part of the process. Instead of quitting, pause and look for solutions. Ask for help, change your plan if needed, and remind yourself of your "why." Be patient and kind with yourself. Progress might be slow some days, but every effort counts.

Reward yourself for your hard work. When you reach a milestone or finish a task, treat yourself to something you enjoy—a favorite snack, a relaxing break, or time with friends. Rewards make the journey more enjoyable and give you something to look forward to.

Staying motivated and accountable is a skill you can build. With the right strategies and support, you will find it easier to maintain high energy and a strong focus. Every step you take brings you closer to your goal, and every day is a new chance to keep moving forward. Remember, you have what it takes to stay on track and succeed—one day, one action at a time.

Overcoming Obstacles in Goal Achievement

No matter how clear your goal is, there will always be obstacles along the way. These obstacles can leave you feeling frustrated, tired, or ready to give up. The truth is that everyone faces challenges when working toward a goal. What matters most is how you handle these challenging moments.

Sometimes, you might lose motivation. Maybe you get bored, feel too busy, or forget why you started. When this happens, return to your original reason for setting the goal. Remind yourself why it is essential. You can also take a short break and come back to your goal with fresh energy.

Other times, life gets in the way. You might get sick, have extra schoolwork or work duties, or face family problems. It is okay to slow down or adjust your plan. If something isn't working, try a different approach. Being flexible and open to change can help you persevere, even if your journey is slower than you had hoped.

Some obstacles come from within. Negative thoughts, such as "I can't do this" or "It's too hard," can lead to self-doubt. When you notice these thoughts, pause and ask, "Is this true?" Remind yourself of the progress you have made and all the steps you have already completed. Celebrate small wins—they demonstrate that you are making progress.

Sometimes you will make mistakes or face setbacks. Perhaps you may miss a deadline or fail to reach a small goal. This is normal. Do not let one mistake stop your progress. Everyone fails sometimes, but what matters is getting back up and trying again. Each mistake is a lesson that can help you improve.

It is also helpful to ask for support when you need it. Discuss your struggles with a friend, family member, or teacher. They can offer advice, encouragement, or listen. You are not alone, and getting help makes you stronger.

Be patient and gentle with yourself. Reaching a goal takes time and effort. Some days will be easy, others will be hard. If you continue, step by step, you will find ways to overcome your obstacles. Every challenge you overcome makes you stronger and brings you closer to success.

Obstacles are a natural part of any journey. By staying flexible, asking for help, and believing in yourself, you can navigate any challenges that come your way and achieve your goals.

CHAPTER 6

Developing Resilience

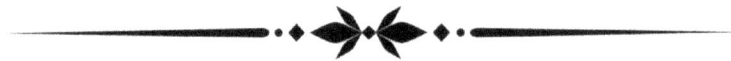

———————— ··◆·◆··————————

Life does not always go as planned. Everyone faces hard times, setbacks, and surprises. What helps you keep going through these challenges is something called resilience. Resilience is your inner strength—the ability to bounce back, adapt, and keep moving forward, even when things get tough. In this chapter, you will learn what resilience means, why it matters, and how you can build it step by step. Developing resilience helps you stay strong during difficult moments and gives you the confidence to face whatever comes your way.

What Is Resilience?

Resilience is the inner strength that helps you navigate difficult times and recover from setbacks. It is what enables you to stand back up when life knocks you down, and keeps you moving forward even when things feel impossible. Resilience does not mean you never feel sad, angry, or worried. Instead, it means that you do not let those feelings stop you from trying again or finding hope.

Think about a time when something did not go the way you wanted. Maybe you failed a test, lost a job, or had a disagreement with a friend. In that moment, you probably felt disappointed or even upset. However, if you were able to calm yourself, create a new plan, or ask for help, you were demonstrating resilience. It is what lets you say, "This is hard, but I will get through it."

Resilience is not something you are born with. It is a skill that you can develop over time, much like building muscle. Each time you deal with a problem, no matter how small, you are teaching yourself to be stronger for the next challenge. This means that even if you do not feel very resilient today, you can become more resilient with practice and effort.

People with resilience do not pretend everything is perfect. They feel pain and sadness like everyone else. What makes them different is how they respond to those feelings. Instead of giving up or blaming themselves, they look for solutions. They might talk to someone they trust, write down their thoughts in a journal, or take a break to clear their mind. They do not let a setback become the end of their journey.

Resilience also means being flexible and open to change. Life is full of surprises, and not everything can be controlled. When things change suddenly, resilient individuals adjust their plans and continue moving forward. They do not get stuck wishing things were different. Instead, they focus on what they can do right now to improve things.

Another part of resilience is hope. Believing that things can improve, even when they are tough, helps you keep moving forward. Hope gives you the strength to try again, even after failure. It enables you to see new possibilities and stay positive, even in the middle of a storm.

Building resilience is not always easy, but there are straightforward ways to get started. You can practice by setting small goals for yourself and persevering when challenges arise. Try to focus on your strengths and the things you have already overcome. Remember the times when you made it through challenging moments in the past. These memories show you that you are stronger than you think.

You can also build resilience by connecting with others. Talking to friends, family, or a mentor can give you support and new ideas for solving problems. Helping others can also make you feel stronger and more hopeful.

Resilience is about believing in yourself, learning from tough times, and never giving up. It is the key to navigating life's challenges and emerging even stronger on the other side. With time and practice, you can build resilience and trust that you can handle whatever comes your way.

Building Resilience in Everyday Life

Building resilience is not just for big life problems. It is something you can practice every single day, even in small moments. When you work on your resilience a little at a time, you become better equipped to handle any challenge, big or small.

One of the best ways to build resilience is to stay positive, even when things do not go your way. Try to look for the good in every situation, no matter how small it may seem. If you miss the bus, you may get extra time to listen to your favorite song. If you make a mistake at work or school, view it as an opportunity to learn something new. By focusing on what you can learn or enjoy, you train your mind to recover more quickly.

Taking care of your body also makes you more resilient. Getting enough sleep, eating healthy foods, and staying active through daily movement help you feel stronger and more resilient to stress. When you feel physically well, it is easier to cope with emotional ups and downs.

Building a routine can also help. When life feels unpredictable, having simple routines gives you something steady to count on. This could mean having a set time for meals, exercise, or quiet time every day. Small routines provide you with comfort and make stressful days feel less overwhelming.

Practicing gratitude is another way to boost resilience. Try writing down three things you are thankful for at the end of each day. They can be as simple as a nice meal, a good conversation, or a sunny afternoon. Focusing on gratitude helps you remember that there are still good things, even when life feels hard.

Learning how to solve problems is a crucial aspect of resilience. When you face a challenge, do not give up right away. Take a moment to think about possible solutions. Break the problem down into smaller pieces and tackle one step at a time. Ask for help if you need it—sometimes, discussing it with a friend or family member can help you see things from a different perspective.

It is also helpful to set small goals and celebrate your progress. Every time you reach a goal, no matter how tiny, you remind yourself that you are capable and moving forward. Even on tough days, a little progress is something to be proud of.

Connecting with others is another key to everyday resilience. Spend time with people who make you feel safe and supported. Share your thoughts and feelings, and listen when others need help as well. Strong relationships help you recover from stress and give you the courage to try new things.

Practice being kind to yourself. When you have a bad day or make a mistake, treat yourself with the same patience you would offer a friend. Remind yourself that everyone has struggles, and it is okay not to be perfect. Give yourself credit for trying and for not giving up.

Practicing these small habits every day, you build resilience that helps you face any challenge. Each positive step, no matter how small, makes you stronger and more ready to handle whatever life brings your way.

Techniques for Bouncing Back

Everyone has tough days—moments when things do not go as planned, and it feels hard to keep going. Bouncing back from setbacks is a key part of resilience. It means you find ways to recover, regain your energy, and get back on track after something difficult happens. Here are some practical and straightforward techniques that can help you bounce back when life gets tough:

First, permit yourself to feel. It is normal to be upset, angry, or disappointed after a setback. Instead of ignoring these feelings, please take a moment to notice them. You should write about what happened or talk to someone you trust. Expressing your feelings helps you work through them and clear your mind for what comes next.

Next, practice self-kindness. When you make a mistake or have a hard day, talk to yourself the way you would speak to a friend. Say things like, "It's okay to make mistakes," or "I'm proud of myself for trying." Avoid harsh self-criticism, as it only makes recovery more difficult.

Take a break and do something you enjoy, even if it's just for a short time. This could be listening to music, going for a walk, reading, or spending time with a pet. Doing something positive helps shift your mood and reminds you that life still has good moments, even when things are hard.

Focus on what you can control. After a setback, it is easy to feel powerless. Instead of worrying about things you cannot change, look for small actions you *can* take. Perhaps you can create a plan to try again, seek advice from someone, or break the problem down into smaller steps. Taking action, no matter how small, gives you a sense of control and helps you feel less stuck.

Learn from the experience. Ask yourself, "What can I take away from this situation?" Even difficult times can teach you valuable lessons. You may discover a new way to solve a problem or learn more about your strengths. Each setback is an opportunity to grow, even if it doesn't feel that way at first.

Set new, realistic goals. If something doesn't work out, try adjusting your plans and setting a new, achievable goal. Breaking your big goals into smaller steps can help you rebuild your confidence and make progress, even after a setback.

Stay connected to people who care about you. Reach out to friends, family, or mentors when you need support. Sharing your struggles and asking for encouragement can make a big difference. Remember, you do not have to bounce back alone.

Be patient with yourself. Recovery takes time. Some days will be better than others. Celebrate every small step you take toward moving forward, and trust that you are becoming stronger with each experience.

Using these techniques, you can recover from setbacks with greater confidence and optimism. Every challenge you face is an opportunity to practice resilience, and each time you get back up, you demonstrate your true strength.

Building Support Systems

Building a strong support system is one of the most effective ways to boost your resilience and help you navigate challenging times. Support systems are the people and groups in your life who listen, encourage, and help you when you need it most. When life feels hard, knowing you are not alone makes every challenge feel lighter and easier to face.

A support system can start with family. Parents, siblings, or other close relatives often know you best. They can offer comfort, advice, and even practical help when you are struggling. It's helpful to let your family know how you're feeling, especially during challenging moments. Having someone to talk to can make a huge difference.

Friends are another key part of your support network. Good friends accept you for who you are, stand by you during hard times, and celebrate your successes. When you share your worries and listen to each other's stories, you feel less alone. Do not hesitate to reach out and tell a friend you need to talk—they are often more willing to help than you might think.

Support does not just come from people you already know. Teachers, coaches, and mentors can also be valuable sources of support. They might have advice, life experience, or just a listening ear when you're unsure about what to do next. If you feel comfortable, let them know what is on your mind. They may have helpful ideas or give you a fresh perspective.

Sometimes, support can be found by joining groups or communities. This could be a school club, a sports team, a community center, or even an online group. Being part of a group helps you meet people who share your interests or who are going through similar challenges. These connections remind you that everyone faces struggles, and you can help each other get through them.

If you find it hard to reach out to others, start small. You do not need to share everything all at once. A simple text, a short conversation, or just spending time with someone you trust can help you feel more connected. Over time, these small moments build into strong, supportive relationships.

It is also essential to be a good support for others. Listen when friends or family need to talk. Offer encouragement and celebrate their progress. When you help others, you strengthen your support network. It feels good to know you are there for each other, no matter what life brings.

Sometimes, professional help is needed. If you feel overwhelmed or unable to cope, it is okay to talk to a counselor, therapist, or doctor. These professionals are trained to help you find solutions and build new skills for resilience.

Everyone needs support sometimes. Asking for help is not a sign of weakness—it is a sign that you care about yourself and want to get stronger. With a strong support system, you can face challenges with more confidence, knowing that, no matter what happens, you are never truly alone.

Practicing Self-Care for Resilience

Taking care of yourself is a key part of building resilience. When you practice self-care, you give your body and mind what they need to stay strong, recover from stress, and keep going, even during tough times. Self-care does not have to be fancy or expensive—it is about making small, healthy choices every day that help you feel your best.

A critical aspect of self-care is maintaining your physical health. Getting enough sleep each night helps your brain and body recover, allowing you to handle challenges with a clear mind. Try to maintain a regular sleep schedule and establish a relaxing bedtime routine, such as reading or listening to calming music, to help you unwind before bed.

Eating healthy foods also supports your resilience. Choose meals that give you steady energy, such as fruits, vegetables, whole grains, and lean proteins. Drinking enough water throughout the day keeps you alert and feeling well. When you fuel your body with nutritious food, you are better equipped to handle both stress and change.

Regular movement is another powerful self-care tool. Exercise doesn't have to mean going to the gym or running long distances. It could be a walk around your neighborhood, dancing to your favorite music, stretching, or playing a sport you enjoy. Moving your body helps release tension and lifts your mood, making it easier to bounce back from difficult moments.

Caring for your mind is just as important as caring for your body. Take time each day to relax and clear your thoughts. This can be achieved through quiet activities such as reading, listening to music, or practicing deep breathing. Mindfulness exercises, such as paying attention to your breath or noticing the sights and sounds around you, can help calm worries and bring you back to the present moment.

Another important self-care habit is setting healthy boundaries. This means saying "no" when you need to, taking breaks, and not trying to do everything at once. Protect your time and energy by focusing on what matters most. It is okay to put yourself first sometimes—this helps you stay balanced and prevents burnout.

Connecting with others is also part of self-care. Spend time with friends or family members who make you feel safe and supported. Talk about your feelings, share your successes and struggles, and listen to those you care about. Strong relationships provide the support you need to recover from setbacks and continue moving forward.

Do not forget to celebrate your efforts and successes, no matter how small they may seem. Take a moment to acknowledge what you've done well each day. This helps build your confidence and reminds you that you are making progress, even on the most challenging days.

If you're having a difficult time, don't hesitate to reach out for extra help. Talking to a counselor, therapist, or support group can give you new tools for self-care and help you feel less alone.

Practicing self-care, you build a strong foundation for resilience. When you treat yourself with kindness and care, you give yourself the strength to face life's challenges, recover from setbacks, and grow even stronger over time.

Real-World Examples of Resilient People

Sometimes the best way to understand resilience is to hear about people who have shown it in real life. Their stories remind us that everyone faces challenges, but with resilience, it is possible to bounce back, grow, and even inspire others.

Consider the story of Ali, a young man who lost his job when the company he worked for closed suddenly. At first, Ali felt hopeless and worried about his future. But instead of giving up, he chose to see this setback as a new beginning. He learned new skills online, sought advice from friends, and eventually found a job that he enjoyed even more than his previous one. Ali's resilience enabled him to turn a challenging situation into an opportunity for growth.

Another example is Maria, a student who struggled in school after moving to a new city. She missed her old friends and struggled to keep up with her new classes. Some days, she wanted to give up. Instead, Maria reached out to her teachers for extra help and joined a school club to make new friends. Slowly, she gained confidence in her studies and began to enjoy her new school. Maria's story demonstrates that resilience is about asking for help, trying new things, and not giving up, even when life seems challenging.

Think of Sara, who faced a serious illness that changed her daily life. At first, she felt scared and unsure about her future. But Sara decided to focus on what she could control — taking care of her health, following her doctors' advice, and staying positive. She kept in touch with loved ones, found comfort in small daily routines, and celebrated every step of progress, no matter how small. Over time, Sara discovered a new strength inside herself and became an inspiration to others facing similar challenges.

There's also Hassan, a father who struggled to support his family after a natural disaster destroyed their home. Even though he felt overwhelmed, Hassan reached out to his community for support, took small jobs to earn money, and worked together with his family to rebuild. Instead of giving in to despair, he showed his children the power of hope, teamwork, and steady effort, even in the face of big problems.

These stories have one thing in common: none of these people gave up when things were hard. They felt sadness, fear, and frustration, but they chose to move forward nonetheless. Sometimes they took tiny steps. Sometimes they asked for help. Most of all, they believed that things could get better, even if the road were long.

Real-life resilience does not mean you are never afraid or upset. It means you keep going, learn from your experiences, and look for new solutions. Every person can be resilient. When you remember the stories of Ali, Maria, Sara, and Hassan, you can find hope and courage for your journey. You, too, can bounce back from challenges and find new strength within yourself.

CHAPTER 7

Building Confidence

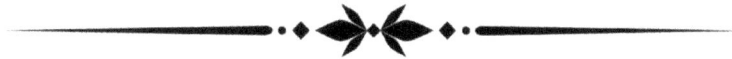

Confidence is believing in yourself and trusting that you can handle whatever comes your way. It is not about being perfect or never feeling afraid. Instead, confidence means knowing your strengths, accepting your weaknesses, and still choosing to try, learn, and grow. In this chapter, you will discover what true confidence looks like, why it matters, and simple ways to build it day by day. When you build your confidence, you open new doors and give yourself the power to chase your dreams, face challenges, and enjoy life with greater courage and joy.

The Psychology of Self-Confidence

Self-confidence is how you feel about your abilities and value. It is shaped by your thoughts, your past experiences, and the messages you hear from others. When you feel confident, you trust yourself to make good choices, try new things, and handle problems—even when you are nervous or unsure.

The way you think about yourself plays a significant role in self-confidence. Positive thoughts like "I can do this" or "I am good at learning new things" help you feel strong inside. On the other hand, negative thoughts such as "I am not smart enough" or "I always fail" can make your confidence drop. Learning to notice and gently change these negative thoughts is one of the best ways to build more self-confidence.

Your experiences also affect your confidence. Each time you try something and succeed—even if it is a small success—your confidence grows. If you make a mistake or something does not work out, it is normal to feel less confident for a while. But if you remind yourself that everyone makes mistakes and that you can learn and improve, your confidence comes back even stronger.

The support you get from others matters, too. Encouragement from family, friends, teachers, or mentors helps you believe in yourself. Sometimes, all it takes is one kind word to help you see your strengths and feel braver.

Self-confidence is not something you are born with or without — it can be built and strengthened over time. By choosing to focus on your strengths, celebrating your progress, and being kind to yourself, you can train your mind to be more confident. This healthy, realistic self-confidence helps you try new things, solve problems, and enjoy life with more happiness and courage.

Identifying Your Strengths

Everyone has strengths, even if you sometimes forget or do not notice them. Your strengths are the skills, talents, and qualities that help you solve problems, connect with others, and make progress in life. When you learn to see and appreciate your strengths, your confidence grows, and you feel more ready to face challenges.

Why Strengths Matter

Knowing your strengths is essential for many reasons. First, it helps you feel proud of who you are. When you remember what you are good at, it is easier to stay positive, even when life is hard. Your strengths give you something to build on. They are your foundation when you want to learn something new or reach a goal.

Understanding your strengths also helps you make better choices. For example, if you are good at listening, you might enjoy jobs or activities where you help others. If you have a creative mind, you could try art, writing, or problem-solving tasks. When you focus on your strengths, you are more likely to enjoy what you do and do it well.

How to Find Your Strengths

Sometimes it is easy to spot your strengths, and sometimes you need to look a little closer. Here are some ways to help you discover what you do well:

Think About What Comes Naturally

Ask yourself, "What do I do easily, even when others find it hard?" You may be good at making friends, solving puzzles, organizing things, or staying calm in challenging situations. Pay attention to the things that feel simple or enjoyable for you.

Notice When You Feel Proud

Think about times when you felt proud of yourself. What were you doing? Were you helping someone, finishing a project, learning something new, or making someone laugh? Moments of pride often point to your natural strengths.

Ask People You Trust

Sometimes other people see your strengths before you do. Ask friends, family members, teachers, or coworkers what they think you are good at. You might be surprised by their answers. They may mention strengths you did not even know you had.

Look at Your Past Successes

Review your achievements, big or small. Did you win an award, complete a challenging task, or get positive feedback? Look for patterns in your successes. You always do well when you work with a team, or you shine when you work alone on creative projects.

Take Strengths Quizzes

Many free online quizzes can help you discover your strengths. These quizzes ask questions about your preferences and habits. They can give you new ideas about what makes you special.

Building on Your Strengths

Once you know your strengths, use them as much as possible. If you are a good listener, offer support to friends. If you love solving problems, volunteer for tasks that need creative thinking. The more you use your strengths, the stronger they become.

At the same time, do not worry if you have areas where you are not as strong. No one is good at everything. Focus on growing your best qualities, and be open to learning new skills as you go.

Turning Weaknesses into Strengths

Sometimes, things you see as weaknesses can become strengths with practice. For example, if you are shy, you might be a careful thinker or a reasonable observer. With time, you can use these qualities to your advantage.

Celebrating Your Unique Strengths

Your strengths are not just about what you can do, but also about who you are. Kindness, honesty, patience, and curiosity are all powerful strengths. Celebrate what makes you unique.

Identifying and building on your strengths, you boost your confidence, achieve more, and enjoy your journey through life. Your strengths are the tools you can use every day to overcome challenges and reach your dreams.

Steps to Build Daily Confidence

Building confidence does not happen overnight. It is a journey made up of small, daily choices and actions. The good news is that anyone can become more confident, no matter where they start. Here are some simple, practical steps you can use each day to boost your confidence and believe in yourself a little more with every sunrise.

1. Start Your Day with Positive Self-Talk

How you speak to yourself matters. Each morning, try to say something kind and encouraging to yourself—even if you do not fully believe it yet. Simple phrases like "I am ready for today," "I can handle what comes my way," or "I am learning and growing" can set a hopeful tone for your day. Over time, positive self-talk can help silence your inner critic and build trust in your abilities.

2. Set Small, Achievable Goals

Big goals are important, but daily confidence is built on small wins. Each morning, set one or two simple goals you know you can reach. It could be as easy as finishing a task at work, making a healthy lunch, or calling a friend. Completing small goals gives you proof that you can follow through, and each success gives you a little boost of confidence to carry into your next challenge.

3. Celebrate Your Successes

Do not wait for something huge to go right before you celebrate yourself. Every small success deserves recognition. At the end of each day, look back and notice what went well, what you finished, and what made you proud. Write your successes in a notebook, share them with a friend, or smile and say, "Well done!" This habit helps your mind focus on progress instead of only noticing what is missing or what went wrong.

4. Practice Good Posture and Body Language

How you carry your body can influence how you feel inside. Stand up straight, relax your shoulders, and look ahead, not down at your feet. Try smiling, even if just for a few seconds. Research shows that standing tall and smiling can make you feel more confident, even when you are nervous.

5. Face Your Fears in Small Steps

Everyone feels afraid sometimes, especially when trying something new. Confidence grows when you face your fears, even in tiny ways. If you are nervous about speaking up, start by saying hello to someone new. If you want to try a new activity, begin by watching or learning about it first. Each small step you take, even if your heart is beating fast, makes the next step easier.

6. Focus on Your Strengths

Spend time doing things you are good at, whether that is drawing, organizing, helping others, or solving problems. When you use your strengths, you feel capable and in control. Remind yourself of these strengths when you start to doubt yourself.

7. Learn from Mistakes Instead of Judging Yourself

Mistakes are a regular part of life and learning. When something goes wrong, try to look for the lesson instead of blaming yourself. Ask, "What can I do differently next time?" By treating mistakes as opportunities to grow, you become less afraid of trying—and much more willing to keep going, even when things do not go as planned.

8. Surround Yourself with Encouraging People

Spend time with people who support you, listen, and lift you. Supportive friends, family, or mentors can remind you of your strengths and help you see the good in yourself. If you find yourself around people who constantly criticize or bring you down, try to limit your time with them and seek out those who make you feel better, not worse.

9. Take Care of Your Body

Your physical health has a significant impact on your confidence. Get enough sleep, eat nourishing foods, drink water, and move your body in ways you enjoy. When you feel strong and healthy, it is easier to believe in yourself and tackle new challenges.

10. Try Something New Each Week

Confidence grows with experience. Challenge yourself to try one new thing every week. It does not have to be big—maybe you taste a new food, learn a new skill, or talk to someone you have not met before. Each new experience helps you discover more about what you are capable of and makes the world feel a little less scary.

11. Practice Gratitude

Take a few minutes each day to notice things you are grateful for, including your qualities and efforts. Gratitude can shift your focus from what you lack to what you already have, helping you feel more content and sure of yourself.

12. Ask for Help When You Need It

Confidence does not mean you do everything alone. Asking for help is a sign of strength. If you are struggling, talk to a friend, family member, or teacher. Everyone needs support sometimes, and getting help can make you feel more confident and less alone.

13. Be Patient with Yourself

Finally, remember that confidence is not built in a day. There will be ups and downs, but every effort you make counts. Be gentle with yourself and celebrate your progress, no matter how slow it seems.

Taking these small, daily steps, you will build absolute, lasting confidence from the inside out. Each new day is another chance to trust yourself a little more, try something new, and become the confident person you want to be.

Facing Your Fears

Fear is something everyone feels at times. It might show up when you have to speak in public, try something new, meet new people, or face a difficult challenge. Sometimes fear can be helpful—it can keep you safe or help you prepare for something important. But if fear holds you back from doing things you want or need to do, it can stop you from growing and reaching your goals.

The first step in facing you fear to notice and name it. Ask yourself, "What am I terrified of?" Maybe you fear making mistakes, being judged by others, failing at a new task, or feeling embarrassed. Writing your fears down can help you see them more clearly and understand where they come from.

Next, remember that you are not alone. Everyone has fears, even the people who look confident on the outside. Many times, the difference between someone who moves forward and someone who stays stuck is not that one is braver than the other—it is simply that one chooses to take action, even while feeling afraid.

Start facing your fears in small, gentle steps. You do not have to jump straight into your biggest fear. Instead, take one tiny step at a time. If you are afraid of talking to new people, start by smiling at someone or saying hello. If public speaking scares you, practice in front of a mirror or record yourself speaking alone in your room. Each small step builds your courage and makes the next step a little easier.

It helps to challenge the thoughts behind your fear. Often, fear is based on "what if" worries that may not be true. Ask yourself, "Is this fear realistic? What's the worst that could happen?" You may realize that even if things do not go perfectly, you will be okay. Remind yourself of times when you were afraid but still managed to succeed, or at least survived and learned something.

Visualize yourself facing your fear and succeeding. Picture yourself giving a good speech, making a new friend, or handling a challenge with confidence. This mental practice can help your brain feel more comfortable and less nervous when you try the real thing.

Permit yourself to feel afraid. It is normal, and it does not mean you are weak or failing. Instead, use fear as a sign that you are stretching and growing. When you do something that scares you, celebrate your courage—even if the result is not perfect.

Ask for support if you need it. Tell a friend or family member about your fears, and let them encourage you. Sometimes, having someone by your side makes all the difference.

After you face a fear, reward yourself. Celebrate your effort, no matter how small the step. Each time you face a fear and move through it, you prove to yourself that you are stronger than you thought.

Facing your fears is not about getting rid of fear altogether. It is about learning to move forward, even when you feel afraid. Each time you take a brave step, you build confidence and show yourself that fear does not have to be in control. Over time, you will find that many things you once feared are no longer so scary—and that you are more capable, courageous, and confident than you ever imagined.

Celebrating Small Wins

When you are working toward a big goal or trying to become more confident, it is natural to focus on the result. You might find yourself thinking only about how far you have to go or worrying that you are not making enough progress. But what helps you move forward is paying attention to the small victories you achieve along the way. Every significant achievement is built on many tiny steps, and each one deserves recognition.

Small wins are those little successes that happen every day. Maybe you finished a task you had been putting off, learned something new, tried something that made you nervous, or stuck to your plan for one more day. These may seem small compared to your final goal, but they matter much more than you might realize. Every time you notice a small win, your mind and body get a burst of positive energy. You feel proud of yourself and start to believe that you really can do what you set out to do. Over time, these feelings of pride and accomplishment build up, creating a habit of noticing what is going well, instead of focusing only on what is missing or what has gone wrong.

One way to make these wins more meaningful is to keep track of them. You could write them down in a notebook or on your phone. At the end of each day or week, take a moment to look back at your list. When you see all the small steps you have taken, it is easier to recognize how much progress you are making, even when it does not feel like much at the time. If you feel comfortable, share your successes with someone you trust, like a friend, family member, or mentor. Telling someone about your small wins makes the moment feel more special and gives you extra encouragement to keep going.

Giving yourself a little reward can also help. After you reach a small milestone, treat yourself to something you enjoy. This could be a favorite snack, some quiet time, or an activity that makes you happy. Rewards make the process of reaching your goal more enjoyable and give you something to look forward to, especially on days when things feel tough.

It is also important to pause and feel proud of what you have done. Sometimes, it is easy to skip right past a small success and jump straight into the next challenge. Instead, give yourself a moment to smile and say, "I did it." Let yourself feel that pride, even if the step was small. These moments help your brain remember how good progress feels, making it easier to try again the next time you are faced with something hard.

When you are feeling discouraged or stuck, look back at your list of small wins. Remind yourself that you have already made progress, even if the journey still feels long. Let those memories encourage you to keep moving forward, no matter how slow it seems. The real magic of building confidence and reaching your goals is not just about crossing the finish line. It is about growing, learning, and enjoying each step along the way. When you take time to celebrate your small wins, you make your journey full of happy moments. This helps you stay positive, recover from setbacks, and keep trying, even when things are difficult.

Every step you take counts. There is no win too small to celebrate. Whether you spoke up in class, finished a workout, tried a new skill, or made it through a hard day, give yourself credit. With every small win, you become stronger, more confident, and more ready to face whatever comes next.

The Role of Positive Relationships

Positive relationships play a decisive role in building confidence and supporting personal growth. When you have people in your life who care about you, encourage you, and celebrate your progress, it becomes much easier to believe in yourself and keep moving forward, even when things get tough. These relationships can be with family, friends, teachers, mentors, or even supportive classmates and coworkers. What matters most is that the people around you treat you with kindness, respect, and understanding.

Good relationships give you a safe place to share your thoughts and feelings. When you feel nervous, stuck, or unsure, being able to talk with someone who listens can help you see things more clearly. They might offer a new perspective or remind you that you are not alone. Sometimes, just knowing that someone cares and is willing to listen is enough to lift your mood and give you the courage to try again.

Positive relationships also give you encouragement to take risks and try new things. When people believe in you and tell you that you can do something, you are more likely to believe it yourself. Their support acts like a safety net, making it easier to step outside your comfort zone.

For example, if you want to join a new club, try out for a team, or speak in front of a group, having someone cheer you on gives you extra confidence to take that leap.

Another way positive relationships help is by celebrating your achievements, no matter how small. When someone notices your progress and says, "I'm proud of you," it feels good and reminds you that your complex work matters. Sharing your successes with others can make each step forward feel even more meaningful. It also gives you a reason to keep trying, even when progress feels slow.

Of course, positive relationships are not only about getting support—they are about giving it, too. When you encourage others, listen to their struggles, and celebrate their wins, you strengthen your bond and create a network of support that goes both ways. Helping someone else can also boost your confidence, as it reminds you of the strengths you have to offer.

Sometimes, building positive relationships means letting go of people who are negative, critical, or unsupportive. If someone constantly brings you down or makes you doubt yourself, it is okay to set boundaries or spend less time with them. Surrounding yourself with people who lift you is not only good for your confidence, but it is also essential for your overall well-being.

It is important to remember that relationships take effort from both sides. Be willing to reach out, offer help, and say thank you. Be honest about your feelings, listen with care, and show appreciation for the people who stand by you. Over time, these actions create trust and make your connections stronger.

When you have positive relationships in your life, you feel more confident, supported, and ready to face whatever challenges come your way. The encouragement and understanding of others remind you that you are never alone on your journey. Whether you are celebrating a win, facing a setback, or simply living day by day, the people who believe in you make every experience richer and more meaningful. Their support helps you become the best version of yourself, one step at a time.

CHAPTER 8

Enhancing Emotional Intelligence

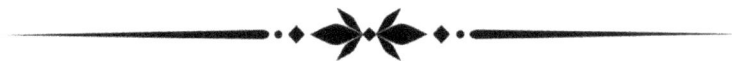

❖◆❖◆❖

Emotional intelligence is the ability to understand and manage your feelings, as well as recognize and respect the feelings of others. It helps you stay calm during stressful times, build better relationships, and make wiser choices every day. In this chapter, you will discover what emotional intelligence means, why it is essential, and how you can strengthen this skill in your own life. Learning to enhance your emotional intelligence will help you feel more confident, connect more deeply with others, and handle life's ups and downs with greater ease.

Understanding Emotional Intelligence (EI)

Emotional intelligence, often called EI or EQ, is an important life skill that affects how we understand ourselves and interact with others. Unlike academic intelligence, which is about solving problems and remembering facts, emotional intelligence is all about recognizing and managing emotions—both your own and those of the people around you. People with strong EI are better at handling stress, communicating, and building positive relationships, which helps them succeed in many parts of life.

Emotional intelligence begins with self-awareness. This means paying attention to your feelings as they happen and being able to name them. For example, you might notice that you are feeling anxious before a test or happy when spending time with friends. The more you understand your own emotions, the easier it is to see how they affect your thoughts and actions. Self-awareness helps you catch yourself before you react out of anger or fear and gives you the chance to choose a better response.

The next part of emotional intelligence is self-management. Once you know what you are feeling, you can start to control how you react. This does not mean you ignore or hide your emotions, but rather that you find healthy ways to deal with them. For instance, if you are feeling stressed, take a few deep breaths, go for a walk, or talk to someone you trust. Self-management also includes staying positive, even during tough times, and bouncing back from setbacks with hope and determination.

Social awareness is another critical piece of EI. This is the ability to notice and understand the feelings of other people. Social awareness means being a good listener, paying attention to body language, and picking up on the emotions in a room. For example, you might notice a friend is quiet and ask if they are okay, or you sense when a group is excited or nervous. Understanding how others feel helps you show empathy, care about, and respect their emotions.

Relationship management is the last part of emotional intelligence. This skill helps you build strong connections with others, handle disagreements, and work well in groups. People with good relationship management skills can communicate, solve problems calmly, and show kindness even when things are difficult. They listen carefully, encourage others, and help bring out the best in everyone around them.

Having high emotional intelligence does not mean you never get upset or make mistakes. It means you are better at understanding what you feel and why, and you can choose how you act. This makes it easier to stay calm under pressure, solve conflicts peacefully, and build trusting relationships.

Emotional intelligence is essential in every part of life. At school, it helps you work well with classmates and manage exam stress. At work, it makes you a better teammate and leader. At home, it strengthens your relationships with family and friends. Even when you are alone, emotional intelligence helps you handle your feelings and make choices that keep you happy and healthy.

The good news is that EI can be developed and improved, no matter your age or background. You can start by paying attention to your feelings, practicing self-control, and being open to the emotions of others. With practice, your emotional intelligence will grow, helping you enjoy better relationships, handle stress, and live a more balanced and confident life.

Self-Awareness and Emotional Regulation

Self-awareness and emotional regulation are two of the most essential parts of emotional intelligence. They work together to help you understand what you are feeling, why you are feeling it, and what you can do about it. When you build these skills, you become better at handling stress, staying calm in challenging situations, and making good decisions — no matter what life throws your way.

Self-awareness starts with noticing your feelings as they happen. This might sound simple, but many people go through the day reacting to their emotions without really thinking about them. For example, you might snap at a friend when you are tired, or feel anxious without realizing you are worried about an upcoming test. Becoming more self-aware means pausing to ask yourself, "What am I feeling right now?" and "Why do I feel this way?" It helps to name your feelings as clearly as possible, such as "I feel frustrated," "I feel excited," or "I feel disappointed." When you can name your emotions, you gain power over them instead of letting them control you.

Journaling is a helpful tool for self-awareness. Writing down your thoughts and feelings at the end of the day can help you spot patterns and triggers. Over time, you start to notice what events, people, or places make you feel specific ways. This insight makes it easier to manage your emotions and plan for tricky situations.

Once you are more aware of your feelings, the next step is emotional regulation — choosing how you react to those feelings. Emotional regulation means you do not let your emotions make decisions for you. Instead, you pause, take a breath, and choose how to respond. For example, if you are angry, instead of yelling or saying something hurtful, you might count to ten, step outside for a few minutes, or talk calmly about what is bothering you. These small actions help you express your emotions in healthy ways and prevent problems from getting worse.

Breathing exercises, mindfulness, and other relaxation techniques are great for managing strong feelings. When you notice stress building, try taking a few slow, deep breaths, focusing on each inhale and exhale. This sends a signal to your brain to calm down and helps you think more clearly. Mindfulness — paying attention to the present moment without judging yourself — also enables you to notice your emotions without getting swept away by them.

Emotional regulation does not mean ignoring your feelings or pretending they are not there. It is about accepting your emotions, permitting yourself to feel them, and then choosing what to do next. Sometimes, that might mean taking a break, talking to someone you trust, or doing something kind for yourself.

Being self-aware and able to regulate your emotions makes it easier to deal with challenges, solve conflicts, and avoid regrets. It also makes you more understanding of other people's feelings, which strengthens your relationships. The more you practice self-awareness and emotional regulation, the more confident and balanced you become.

No one gets it right all the time. Learning to be aware of and manage your feelings is a lifelong journey. Be patient with yourself and celebrate your progress. With time, you will find it easier to stay calm under pressure, make thoughtful choices, and enjoy stronger, healthier connections with others.

Building Empathy

Empathy is the ability to understand and share the feelings of another person. It is a powerful part of emotional intelligence because it helps you connect with others in an honest and caring way. When you are empathetic, you can put yourself in someone else's shoes and imagine what they might be thinking or feeling. This skill not only helps build strong friendships and relationships but also makes you a kinder, more understanding person.

Building empathy begins with listening. When someone talks to you about their feelings or a problem they are facing, try to give them your full attention. Put away distractions, look them in the eye, and focus on their words. Sometimes, people do not need advice—they want someone to listen and understand. When you listen without interrupting or judging, you show that you respect their experience and care about what they are going through.

It also helps to notice body language and tone of voice. Sometimes people are not ready or able to say precisely how they feel with words, but their actions or expressions can give you clues. If a friend seems quiet or withdrawn, or if they look worried or sad, it may be a sign that something is wrong. Asking gentle questions like, "Are you okay?" or "Do you want to talk about it?" can open the door for them to share more.

Empathy means not rushing to judge or give advice right away. Instead, try to understand their point of view, even if it is different from your own. You might say, "That sounds tough," or "I can see why you would feel that way." These simple words can be comforting and let the other person know you are on their side.

Another way to build empathy is to imagine how you would feel if you were in the other person's situation. Ask yourself, "How would I feel if that happened to me?" or "What would I want someone to say or do if I were in their shoes?" This kind of thinking helps you respond with kindness and patience.

Sharing your feelings can also help build empathy, as long as you do it in a way that does not take the focus away from the other person. For example, you might say, "I've felt nervous before a big test, too," or "I know what it's like to feel left out." Sharing these experiences lets others know they are not alone, but remember to keep the conversation centered on their needs.

Empathy is not just about difficult moments. It also means sharing in someone's happiness and success. Celebrate their good news, offer praise, and show excitement for their achievements. Being genuinely happy for others builds trust and strengthens your relationships.

Practicing empathy every day helps you become a better friend, partner, and team member. It makes it easier to handle disagreements and solve problems because you understand where the other person is coming from. Empathy also makes you feel more connected to the people around you, which can bring more joy and meaning to your life.

Building empathy takes time and practice, but every effort makes a difference. The more you listen, imagine, and care, the easier it becomes to connect with others genuinely and compassionately. Empathy is one of the most important skills you can have for a happier, healthier, and more successful life.

Tools for Better Social Skills

Good social skills help you connect with others, build lasting friendships, and feel more comfortable in social situations. These skills are not just for outgoing people—anyone can learn and improve them with a bit of practice. When you use the right tools, you feel more confident talking, listening, and working together with people from all walks of life.

One of the best tools for better social skills is learning how to be a good listener. This means focusing on what the other person is saying instead of thinking about what you want to say next. Try to make eye contact, nod, and give minor signs that you are interested. Let the person finish their thoughts before you reply. Being a good listener shows respect and helps you understand others better, making conversations feel more natural and meaningful.

Another helpful skill is asking open-ended questions. Instead of questions that can be answered with a simple yes or no, try asking questions that invite people to share more about themselves. For example, instead of asking, "Did you have a good weekend?" you might say, "What did you do over the weekend?" Open-ended questions keep conversations going and show that you care about the other person's thoughts and experiences.

Learning to give compliments is also essential. Honest, kind compliments can make someone's day and help build a positive atmosphere. Focus on something specific, like "I liked your presentation," or "You did a great job organizing the event." When you notice and appreciate what others do well, it strengthens your relationships and encourages them to do the same for you.

Being aware of your body language is another helpful tool. Smile, stand or sit up straight, and use gestures that match your words. Positive body language makes you appear more open, friendly, and confident. At the same time, please pay attention to other people's body language so you can notice how they are feeling.

Practicing empathy also helps you get along with others. Try to see things from their point of view, even if you disagree. Respond with kindness and patience, especially during disagreements. Empathy helps you handle misunderstandings and makes it easier to solve problems together.

Another essential tool is learning how to express yourself clearly and honestly. Use "I" statements to share your feelings, like "I feel happy when we spend time together," or "I feel frustrated when I am not heard." Clear communication helps avoid confusion and lets others know how you truly feel.

It is also helpful to practice handling rejection or awkward moments. Not every conversation or friendship will go perfectly, and that is okay. If something feels uncomfortable, take a deep breath, stay polite, and remember that everyone makes mistakes or feels awkward sometimes. Each experience is a chance to learn and grow.

To say thank you and show appreciation. Gratitude is a simple way to strengthen your social bonds and leave a good impression. When you show others that you value them, you make it more likely that they will want to spend time with you again.

Improving your social skills is a lifelong process, but every effort brings you closer to being more comfortable and confident with others. By practicing these tools, you build better relationships, enjoy richer conversations, and open yourself up to new opportunities and friendships throughout your life.

EI at Work and Home

Emotional intelligence, or EI, is just as critical at work and home as it is in any other part of life. In both places, you are around other people, face challenges, and sometimes deal with stress or disagreements. When you use your emotional intelligence skills, you make life smoother, build stronger relationships, and solve problems more easily.

At work, EI helps you communicate clearly and work well with others. If you are on a team, being able to listen, understand different points of view, and respect everyone's ideas is a significant advantage. When you pay attention to your feelings, you notice when you are stressed or frustrated and can take a break or talk things through calmly instead of letting emotions get out of control. If you see a coworker is upset or having a hard day, showing empathy and offering a kind word can make a huge difference. This not only builds trust but also makes the workplace more positive for everyone.

EI is also helpful when dealing with feedback or criticism at work. Instead of taking things personally or getting defensive, you can use your self-awareness to listen, consider what you can learn, and respond politely. This shows that you care about improving and that you are mature enough to handle tough conversations. People with strong EI are often chosen for leadership roles because they can handle stress, motivate others, and solve conflicts fairly.

At home, emotional intelligence makes your relationships with family and loved ones warmer and more supportive. When you understand your own emotions, you are less likely to lose your temper or say things you regret. If you notice you are tired, anxious, or upset, you can tell your family how you feel in a calm way. This makes it easier to ask for help or get some quiet time when you need it.

Listening and showing empathy at home is just as crucial as at work. When a family member is sad, excited, or worried, taking the time to listen and support them helps everyone feel closer. Even simple things, like asking how someone's day went or saying thank you for something kind they did, can make your home feel happier and safer.

Conflicts and disagreements happen at home just like anywhere else. Using EI means staying calm, listening to each other, and trying to solve problems together. You can practice using "I feel" statements instead of blaming, and work on finding solutions that work for everyone. Over time, this builds trust and keeps your family strong, even when times are tough.

Balancing work and home life can be stressful, but EI helps you handle pressure in healthy ways. Instead of letting stress from work spill over into your home life, you can practice self-care, set boundaries, and ask for support when you need it. If you are feeling overwhelmed, talking about your feelings with someone you trust can help you find new solutions and feel less alone.

In both work and home settings, EI helps you understand yourself, connect with others, and build relationships based on respect and kindness. These skills make every day smoother and more enjoyable. With practice, emotional intelligence becomes a natural part of how you think, act, and interact—helping you succeed and feel happier wherever you are.

Practices to Strengthen EI

Strengthening your emotional intelligence (EI) is something anyone can do, no matter their age or background. With practice and patience, you can become more aware of your feelings, manage your emotions better, and improve your relationships at home, work, and everywhere in between. Here are some simple, every day practices to help you build stronger EI.

Start by making time for self-reflection. Each day, set aside a few minutes to think about how you felt and acted during the day. Ask yourself questions like, "What emotions did I feel today?" and "How did I react when something made me happy, sad, or upset?" Writing your answers in a journal can help you spot patterns over time and learn more about what triggers your emotions. The more you notice your feelings, the easier it is to understand and manage them.

Practice pausing before reacting. When you notice a strong emotion, whether it's anger, excitement, or fear, take a deep breath and wait for a moment. Give yourself a chance to think about what you want to say or do before you react. This slight pause can help you avoid saying things you regret and give you time to choose a calmer, more thoughtful response.

Work on your listening skills. When someone is talking to you, please give them your full attention. Put away your phone or any other distractions, make eye contact, and show that you care about what they are saying. Listen not just to their words, but also to their tone of voice and body language. Try to understand how they feel, and ask questions if you're not sure. Good listening builds trust and helps you connect with others more deeply.

Show empathy whenever you can. Try to imagine how someone else might be feeling, especially during disagreements or stressful times. You do not have to agree with them, but you can show that you care by saying things like, "That sounds tough," or "I'm here if you want to talk." Small acts of empathy help people feel valued and supported, making your relationships stronger and kinder.

Practice expressing your feelings in healthy ways. Instead of hiding your emotions or letting them explode, try to talk about them honestly and calmly. Use "I feel" statements to share what's going on inside, like "I feel frustrated when meetings run late," or "I feel happy when we spend time together." Clear communication helps others understand you better and builds respect on both sides.

Pay attention to stress and take care of yourself. Emotional intelligence includes recognizing when you need a break, asking for help, or saying no to extra tasks when you feel overwhelmed. Find healthy ways to manage stress, like exercise, spending time in nature, listening to music, or practicing deep breathing. Self-care keeps your emotions in balance and helps you recharge.

Be open to feedback from others. Sometimes, the people around you can see things about your behavior or emotions that you might miss. If someone gives you advice or shares how your actions made them feel, listen with an open mind. Feedback is a chance to learn and grow, not something to fear.

Keep practicing kindness and patience with yourself. No one is perfect, and building emotional intelligence is a lifelong journey. Celebrate your progress, forgive yourself for mistakes, and keep trying to do a little better each day.

Practicing these habits, you will strengthen your emotional intelligence over time. The result is better relationships, more self-control, and greater happiness—both for yourself and for everyone you interact with.

CHAPTER 9

Improving Communication

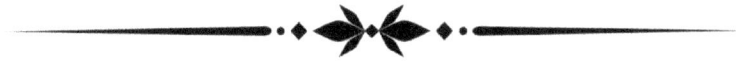

———————◆◆◆◆———————

Communication is more than just talking—it is how we share our ideas, feelings, and needs with others. Good communication helps us build trust, solve problems, and create strong connections at home, at work, and in everyday life. In this chapter, you will discover why communication matters so much, what makes someone a good communicator, and how you can practice simple skills to express yourself clearly and listen with understanding. By improving your communication, you can avoid misunderstandings, build better relationships, and feel more confident in every conversation.

The Importance of Communication

Communication is at the heart of almost everything we do. It is how we connect with others, share our thoughts and feelings, and make sense of the world around us. Whether you are talking with family, working on a project with classmates or coworkers, or making new friends, communication plays a vital role in every relationship. Without clear and honest communication, misunderstandings can easily happen, feelings can get hurt, and problems can grow instead of being solved.

One reason communication is so important is that it helps build trust between people. When you are open and transparent about what you think and how you feel, others know they can rely on you. Trust grows stronger when people feel safe to share their own thoughts and know they will be listened to without judgment. This is true at home, at school, at work, and in friendships. The more you communicate openly and respectfully, the stronger your relationships become.

Good communication is also the key to working together and solving problems. If you are part of a team, you need to share ideas, listen to each other's opinions, and make plans together. When everyone understands what is expected and what the goal is, it is much easier to stay focused and get things done. If a problem or disagreement comes up, honest communication lets everyone express their point of view and work toward a solution that feels fair. This makes group work more enjoyable and successful.

Being able to communicate well helps you express your needs and set healthy boundaries. For example, if you feel overwhelmed with school or work, telling someone how you feel and what you need makes it more likely that you will get support. If you are unhappy with the way someone treats you, good communication helps you stand up for yourself in a calm, respectful way. It gives you the confidence to say yes when something feels right and no when it does not.

Communication is not just about talking—it is also about listening. When you listen carefully to others, you show that you respect them and value their feelings. Listening can help you learn new things, understand different points of view, and avoid making quick judgments. It can even help prevent arguments before they start, because people feel heard and understood.

In daily life, strong communication makes everything smoother. At home, it helps families plan together, support one another, and solve minor problems before they become big ones. With friends, good communication makes it easier to share joys and worries, make plans, and build memories together. At work or in school, it lets you work well with others, ask questions, and give feedback in a helpful way.

Communication also boosts your self-confidence. When you can share your thoughts clearly and listen with understanding, you feel more sure of yourself in all kinds of situations. You are more likely to speak up in class, at meetings, or during meaningful conversations. This makes it easier to make friends, ask for what you need, and step into new opportunities.

Most importantly, communication is a skill you can practice and improve at any age. It takes time and effort, but every conversation is a chance to learn. By focusing on both speaking and listening, being honest and respectful, and paying attention to how your words affect others, you become a better communicator—and a stronger, more caring person.

Communication is much more than just talking. It is a bridge that connects you with the people in your life, helps you solve problems, and gives you the tools to build the relationships and life you want. By working on your communication skills, you can improve every part of your life and make every day a little brighter.

Verbal and Non-Verbal Communication

Communication is not just about the words you say. It also includes the way you tell them and the signals your body gives while you are talking. Verbal communication is the use of spoken or written words to share your thoughts, ideas, or feelings. Non-verbal communication is everything you express without words, like your facial expressions, body language, gestures, tone of voice, and even the way you make eye contact.

Verbal communication is essential because it lets you share information clearly and directly. When you use words, you can ask questions, tell stories, give directions, or explain how you feel. Good verbal communication means choosing words that are easy to understand and using a tone that matches your message. If you are excited, your voice might be lively and happy. If you are serious, your tone may be calm and steady. Speaking clearly and at the right speed helps others follow what you are saying. When you listen to someone else, paying attention to their words and asking questions if you do not understand shows respect and helps avoid confusion.

Non-verbal communication can sometimes be more potent than words. Your body often shows how you really feel, sometimes without you even noticing. For example, if you are nervous, you might fidget or avoid eye contact. If you are happy, you might smile, stand tall, or laugh. When someone is upset but says they are "fine," their body language may tell a different story. People often believe what they see more than what they hear, so if your words and your body language do not match, others may feel confused or think you are not telling the truth.

Gestures, like waving, nodding, or giving a thumbs-up, can add meaning to your words or help you communicate even when you do not speak the same language. Facial expressions—like smiling, frowning, or raising your eyebrows—give clues about how you are feeling. Eye contact is another important signal; looking someone in the eyes shows you are paying attention, while looking away too much might make you seem unsure or distracted.

The tone and volume of your voice are also part of non-verbal communication. Saying "I'm sorry" in a gentle, caring voice means something different from saying it in a cold or rushed way. When you speak softly, it can show kindness or calm. When your voice is loud and sharp, it can sound angry or excited. By paying attention to your tone, you can help others understand your true feelings.

The space between you and another person—sometimes called "personal space"—also sends a message. Standing too close can make people feel uncomfortable, while standing too far away can seem unfriendly. Finding a comfortable distance shows respect and helps people feel safe.

Understanding both verbal and non-verbal communication can help you express yourself better and read other people's feelings more accurately. When you talk to someone, try to notice not just what they say, but how they say it and what their body is doing. This can help you spot when someone is confused, upset, or excited, and adjust your own words or actions to match the situation.

Practicing good communication means being aware of both your words and your actions. The more you pay attention to these signals, the easier it is to connect with others, avoid misunderstandings, and build trust in every conversation. By combining strong verbal and non-verbal skills, you can make sure your message is clear and your relationships are strong.

Active Listening Skills

Listening is one of the most essential parts of good communication, but it is also something people often overlook. Many times, people focus on what they want to say next instead of really hearing what the other person is saying. Active listening is a special way of listening that helps you understand, connect, and respond better in every conversation.

Active listening means giving your full attention to the person speaking. This starts with putting away distractions—turn off your phone or look away from the TV so you can focus just on the conversation. Make eye contact to show you are interested and nod your head or smile to encourage the speaker to keep talking. These small actions let the other person know you value what they have to say.

Another key part of active listening is using your body language. Lean in a little when someone is talking to you and face them directly. Avoid crossing your arms or looking around the room, which might make you seem bored or impatient. Open and relaxed body language makes you look approachable and helps the speaker feel comfortable sharing their thoughts.

While listening, do your best not to interrupt or jump in with your own opinions. Sometimes, you might feel tempted to finish the other person's sentences or give advice right away, but it is better to let them speak until they are finished. Give them time to explain, even if you already think you know what they are going to say. This shows respect and helps you fully understand their message.

As you listen, pay close attention to both the words and the feelings behind them. Notice the speaker's tone of voice and facial expressions. Sometimes, what a person says does not match how they really feel. For example, they might say, "I'm fine," but their voice sounds sad or their face looks worried. Picking up on these clues can help you respond with kindness and empathy.

To show that you are listening, try repeating back what you heard in your own words. You might say, "So, you're feeling stressed about your new job?" or "It sounds like you're excited about your trip." This is called reflecting, and it lets the speaker know you understand them. If you are not sure what they mean, ask gentle questions like, "Can you tell me more?" or "How did that make you feel?" Asking questions shows curiosity and helps keep the conversation going.

Giving feedback is another part of active listening. Feedback does not mean criticizing or judging; it means offering your thoughts in a supportive way. If you have advice or an idea to share, wait until the person is done talking and then ask if they would like to hear it. Respect their answer if they want to be heard.

Sometimes, active listening means just being there without needing to fix anything. People often feel better simply because someone took the time to listen. It builds trust and can even strengthen your relationship.

Active listening takes practice, but every effort makes a difference. When you listen actively, you make others feel valued and understood, which makes them more likely to listen to you in return. These skills help you avoid misunderstandings, solve problems peacefully, and create stronger, more positive connections with everyone you meet.

Making active listening a habit, you not only improve your communication skills but also become a better friend, family member, coworker, and leader. Every conversation is a chance to show care and respect, one listening ear at a time.

Assertiveness without Aggression

Being assertive means speaking up for yourself in a way that is honest, respectful, and calm. It is a skill that helps you share your thoughts, feelings, and needs without putting others down or causing unnecessary conflict. Assertiveness is not the same as aggression. When you are aggressive, you try to control, blame, or hurt others with your words or actions. Assertiveness, on the other hand, is about expressing yourself clearly while still respecting the rights and feelings of those around you.

One of the first steps to being assertive is knowing what you want or need. Take time to think about your feelings and beliefs before you speak. Ask yourself, "What do I want in this situation?" and "How can I say this honestly without hurting anyone?" When you are clear about your own needs, it is much easier to communicate them confidently.

Assertive communication uses simple, direct language. Instead of hinting or hoping someone will guess what you need, say it calmly and politely. Use "I" statements to take responsibility for your feelings and avoid blaming others. For example, say, "I feel overwhelmed when meetings run late," instead of, "You always make meetings run too long." This keeps the conversation focused on your feelings and helps prevent the other person from getting defensive.

Body language is also essential in assertive communication. Stand or sit up straight, look the other person in the eye, and speak with a steady voice. Try to stay relaxed and open rather than tense or angry. Your posture and tone can help show that you mean what you say and that you are not trying to start a fight.

Listening is a key part of assertiveness. After you express your needs or opinions, give the other person a chance to respond. Listen carefully, even if you disagree. Respect their point of view and try to find common ground. Assertiveness is about creating a conversation, not giving orders or shutting people down.

Sometimes, being assertive means saying no. If someone asks you to do something that feels wrong, too stressful, or just not right for you, it is okay to refuse politely. You can say, "No, thank you," or "I'm not able to help with that right now." You do not need to apologize for having boundaries or for taking care of yourself. Saying no with respect is a healthy way to protect your time, energy, and well-being.

Assertiveness can feel uncomfortable at first, especially if you are used to staying quiet or going along with what others want. It takes practice, but each time you stand up for yourself, it gets a little easier. Remember that you are allowed to have your own opinions and needs, just like everyone else.

Sometimes, people may not agree with you or may react strongly. Stay calm and polite, even if the other person becomes upset. If things get heated, take a deep breath, pause, or ask to continue the conversation later. Assertiveness is not about winning an argument; it is about standing up for yourself and creating respect on both sides.

Practicing assertiveness without aggression, you build stronger relationships and more self-confidence. You show others that you respect yourself and them. Over time, you will find that people are more likely to listen to you, trust you, and treat you with respect in return. Assertiveness is a powerful tool for healthy communication, problem-solving, and personal growth.

Navigating Difficult Conversations

Difficult conversations are a part of life. Everyone has to face them from time to time, whether it is telling someone you disagree, sharing bad news, setting a boundary, or talking about a problem that needs to be fixed. These conversations can feel stressful, but learning how to handle them in a calm and respectful way can make a big difference in your relationships and your peace of mind.

The first step in navigating a difficult conversation is to prepare yourself. Please take a moment to think about what you want to say and why it is essential. Try to understand your feelings about the situation and what outcome you hope for. If you are upset, take some deep breaths or wait until you feel calmer before starting the conversation. Being clear-headed helps you stay focused and avoid saying things you do not mean.

When the time comes to talk, choose a good place and time for the conversation. Find somewhere private and quiet where you both can feel comfortable. Avoid starting difficult conversations when you or the other person is tired, hungry, or distracted. A calm environment helps both people feel safe to share and listen.

Use clear, honest, and gentle language when you begin. Try to use "I" statements to express your feelings and needs, like "I feel worried about our deadlines," instead of "You never finish your work on time." This keeps the focus on your experience instead of blaming the other person, which can help prevent defensiveness.

Listening is just as essential as talking during a difficult conversation. Give the other person time to share their side. Listen with an open mind and try not to interrupt. Sometimes, repeating back what you heard in your own words can show that you understand, such as "So, you're feeling stressed about the changes at work?" This helps clear up confusion and builds trust.

Stay as calm as possible, even if the conversation becomes emotional. If you feel yourself getting upset, pause for a moment or take a few slow breaths. If things get too heated, ask for a break and agree to continue talking later. It is better to pause and cool off than to say something you might regret.

During the conversation, try to find common ground or a solution that works for both sides. Ask questions like, "What do you think we can do to fix this?" or "How can we move forward from here?" Working together to solve the problem builds respect and makes it easier to move on after the conversation ends.

Remember, you do not have to agree on everything. The goal of a difficult conversation is not to "win" but to understand each other and find a way to move forward. Even if you do not reach a perfect solution, being honest, respectful, and willing to listen makes a big difference.

After the conversation, take a moment to care for yourself. Difficult talks can be draining. Spend some time doing something calming or enjoyable, and remind yourself that having these conversations is a sign of strength and maturity.

Navigating difficult conversations is not easy, but with practice, it gets better. Each time you handle a tough talk with care, you build more trust, confidence, and understanding in your relationships. You show yourself and others that problems can be faced and solved with kindness, respect, and a little courage.

Improving Communication in Relationships

Good communication is the foundation of any strong relationship, whether it's with family, friends, a partner, or coworkers. When you communicate well, you create trust, avoid misunderstandings, and help everyone feel heard and respected. Improving communication in your relationships does not mean you will never have disagreements. Still, it makes it much easier to work through problems together and enjoy the good times even more.

One of the best ways to improve communication is to make time for honest conversations. This means setting aside moments where you can give each other your full attention without distractions from phones, television, or other interruptions. Even just a few minutes of focused conversation each day can make a big difference in how connected you feel.

Listening is at the heart of good communication. Practice truly listening to what the other person is saying, instead of thinking about what you want to say next. Let them finish speaking before you respond, and show you are interested by nodding, making eye contact, or asking gentle questions. When someone feels listened to, they are more likely to open up and share honestly.

Be honest and transparent about your thoughts and feelings. If something is bothering you, try to share it calmly and respectfully, using "I" statements such as "I feel hurt when plans change without notice" instead of blaming or accusing. Sharing your feelings honestly builds trust and prevents misunderstandings from growing.

It also helps to check in regularly, even when things are going well. Ask how the other person is feeling, what is on their mind, or if there's anything they want to talk about. This shows you care and want to stay connected, not just during tough times but all the time.

Pay attention to your body language and tone of voice. Sometimes, how you say something matters as much as the words you use. A warm tone, a gentle smile, or an open posture can make your message feel more caring and safe. If you are upset, take a moment to calm down before you talk, so your words and actions match what you truly want to say.

When conflicts do come up, try to solve them together. Instead of trying to win an argument, focus on finding a solution that works for both of you. Listen to each other's point of view, look for areas of agreement, and be willing to compromise when possible. If things get too heated, it is okay to take a break and return to the conversation when you both feel calmer.

Celebrate the good moments in your relationship. Saying thank you, sharing compliments, or simply spending time together helps strengthen your bond and makes it easier to communicate when things are hard.

Be patient with yourself and with others. Communication is a skill that takes time to develop, and everyone makes mistakes sometimes. What matters is being willing to keep trying, to apologize when you get it wrong, and to forgive and move forward.

Practicing these habits, you can improve communication in any relationship. Over time, you will find it easier to share your thoughts and feelings, listen with empathy, and solve problems as a team. Good communication helps every relationship grow stronger, happier, and more supportive, making life better for everyone involved.

CHAPTER 10

Managing Stress

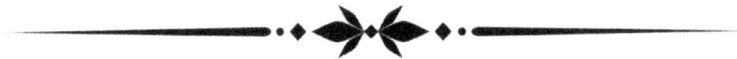

—— ••◆►◆•• ——

Stress is something everyone experiences at different times in life. It can come from school, work, relationships, or unexpected events. While stress is a regular part of life, too much of it can make you feel tired, worried, or overwhelmed. The good news is that you can learn healthy ways to manage stress and protect your mind and body. In this chapter, you will discover what stress is, how it affects you, and practical tips for handling it. By learning to manage stress, you can stay calm, focused, and enjoy life more, even when things get tough.

The Science of Stress

Stress is your body's natural reaction to challenges or demands. It is something everyone feels from time to time, whether the stress comes from a big exam, changes at work, problems at home, or even exciting events like moving to a new place. Understanding how stress works can help you manage it better and stay healthy.

When you face a stressful situation, your brain quickly senses that something needs your attention. It sends signals to your body to get ready for action. This is called the "fight or flight" response. Your heart beats faster, your muscles tense up, and your breathing becomes quicker. These changes are meant to help you react quickly and stay safe. For example, if you were in real danger, this response would help you run away or protect yourself. Even today, the fight or flight response enables you to focus and get through challenging or essential moments.

Not all stress is bad. Sometimes, stress gives you the energy and focus to do your best, like studying for a big test, meeting a deadline, or performing in a game. This kind of short-term stress usually goes away when the challenge is over, and your body returns to normal. It is called "acute stress," and it can be helpful in small doses.

The problem happens when stress lasts too long or feels too strong. When your body stays in a state of stress for days or weeks, it is called "chronic stress." Chronic stress can make you feel tired, anxious, or easily upset. It can also lead to headaches, trouble sleeping, stomach problems, and a weaker immune system. Over time, too much stress can make it harder to think clearly and can even affect your heart and other organs.

Your thoughts and feelings play a big part in how much stress you feel. If you think you cannot handle a situation, or you expect things to go wrong, your brain will send out more stress signals. On the other hand, if you believe you can cope or you find ways to relax, your body calms down more quickly.

Everyone feels stress differently, and what stresses one person may not bother another at all. Some people feel stress in their bodies, with aches or tiredness. Others think more of their emotions, with worry or sadness. That is why it is essential to notice your signs of stress and learn what helps you relax.

Understanding the science of stress gives you the power to handle it in healthy ways. By paying attention to your body, changing negative thoughts, and practicing calming techniques, you can lower your stress and protect your health. Remember, stress is a regular part of life, but with the right tools, you can keep it from taking over and keep moving forward with strength and confidence.

Identifying Stress Triggers

One of the best ways to manage stress is to understand what causes it in your life. These causes are called stress triggers. A stress trigger is anything that sets off feelings of worry, frustration, or tension. Triggers can be big or small, and they are different for everyone. When you learn to spot your stress triggers, you can prepare for them or find new ways to cope.

Some everyday stress triggers include things like pressure at work or school, arguments with family or friends, health problems, financial worries, or significant life changes like moving or starting a new job. Even happy events, such as planning a wedding or having a baby, can bring stress because they involve change and new responsibilities.

Daily hassles are also everyday stress triggers. These are the small things that build up over time, like running late, traffic jams, noisy environments, too much screen time, or not getting enough sleep. If you ignore these minor stressors, they can add up and make you feel overwhelmed.

Sometimes, stress triggers come from the way you think about situations. If you tend to expect the worst or feel like you must be perfect all the time, you may create extra stress for yourself. Comparing yourself to others, worrying about things you cannot control, or being too hard on yourself are all mental habits that can trigger stress.

To identify your stress triggers, start by paying close attention to when you feel stressed. Notice what is happening around you, what you are thinking, and how your body feels. Are your muscles tight? Is your heart beating fast? Do you feel nervous, angry, or sad? Try keeping a stress diary for a week or two. Write down each time you notice yourself feeling stressed, what was going on, and how you responded. Patterns may start to appear that help you see your primary triggers.

Talking to someone you trust about your stress can also help. Sometimes, others can see patterns that you miss. A friend, family member, or counselor can help you figure out which situations, people, or thoughts tend to set off your stress. Together, you can brainstorm ways to deal with these triggers in a healthier way.

Once you know your primary stress triggers, you can make a plan to handle them better. You can avoid some triggers or prepare for them ahead of time. For those you cannot change, you can practice calming techniques or adjust how you think about the situation. With practice, you will find that you feel more in control and less overwhelmed by stress.

Identifying stress triggers is an essential step in building a healthier, more peaceful life. When you understand what causes your stress, you have the power to make changes, ask for support, and protect your well-being every day.

Short-Term Coping Techniques

When stress shows up, it can feel overwhelming, but there are many simple techniques you can use to calm down quickly and get back on track. Short-term coping techniques are strategies you can use right away, in the moment, to manage your stress and find relief. These techniques help you pause, catch your breath, and clear your mind so you can handle the situation more calmly.

One of the most effective short-term coping techniques is deep breathing. When you feel stressed, your breathing often becomes shallow and fast. By taking slow, deep breaths, you signal your body to relax. Try this: breathe in slowly through your nose for a count of four, hold for a moment, and then breathe out slowly through your mouth for a count of four. Repeat this several times. You will likely feel your heart rate slow, and your muscles begin to relax.

Another helpful technique is grounding yourself in the present moment. Sometimes, stress makes your mind race with worries about the past or future. To ground yourself, focus on what is happening right now. Notice five things you can see, four things you can touch, three things you can hear, two things you can smell, and one thing you can taste. This exercise brings your attention back to the present and helps stop anxious thoughts.

Physical activity, even just for a few minutes, can quickly reduce stress. If you feel tense, try taking a brisk walk, stretching, or moving your body in a way that feels good. Exercise helps release stress hormones and produces endorphins, the body's natural mood boosters.

Sometimes, stepping outside for fresh air or changing your environment, even briefly, can make a big difference in how you feel.

Talking to someone you trust can also help you cope with stress in the moment. Call or text a friend, family member, or counselor and share what you are feeling. Sometimes, just hearing a kind voice or getting advice from someone else can help you feel less alone and more supported.

Taking a break is another valuable coping technique. Step away from the stressful situation, and do something you enjoy or find calming. Listen to your favorite music, read a few pages of a book, or watch a funny video. Even a short break gives your mind time to reset.

Some people find that writing down their thoughts and feelings in a journal helps them process stress. Try jotting down what is bothering you, how you feel, and what you might do next. Getting your worries out on paper can make them feel less heavy.

Try positive self-talk. Remind yourself that stress is temporary and that you have overcome hard things before. Say to yourself, "I can handle this," or "This feeling will pass." Encouraging words can boost your mood and give you the strength to keep going.

Coping techniques do not make problems disappear, but they help you handle stress in the moment so you can think more clearly and make better choices. By practicing these skills, you will be better prepared to manage stressful situations whenever they arise, keeping your mind and body healthier and more at ease.

Long-Term Stress Management Strategies

While short-term coping techniques help you calm down quickly, long-term stress management is about building habits that keep your mind and body healthy every day. These strategies do not just help you when stress hits — they make you more resilient and better able to handle life's ups and downs in the future.

One of the most important long-term strategies is taking care of your body. Regular exercise, even something as simple as walking or stretching, helps release tension, lift your mood, and keep stress hormones in check. Try to find an activity you enjoy and make it a part of your weekly routine. Good nutrition also matters. Eating balanced meals with plenty of fruits, vegetables, and whole grains gives your body the fuel it needs to handle stress. Do your best to avoid too much caffeine, sugar, and junk food, as these can make stress feel worse.

Getting enough sleep is another key part of long-term stress management. When you are rested, you are better able to think, manage your emotions, and face challenges. Create a calming bedtime routine, go to bed at the same time each night, and keep your sleeping space quiet and comfortable. If you have trouble sleeping, gentle stretches, deep breathing, or reading a book can help you unwind.

Building strong, supportive relationships is also essential for managing stress over time. Make time for friends and family who make you feel safe and valued. Please share your thoughts and listen to theirs. Ask for help when you need it, and offer support when others need you. Knowing you are not alone makes life's challenges easier to face.

Managing your time wisely is another helpful strategy. Try using a planner or calendar to organize your day. Break big tasks into smaller steps, set realistic goals, and permit yourself to say no to extra commitments when you feel overloaded. By planning, you reduce last-minute rush and feel more in control.

Practicing relaxation and mindfulness every day is a powerful way to build long-term resilience. Take a few minutes each day to breathe deeply, meditate, or sit quietly and notice your thoughts and feelings. Mindfulness helps you stay calm, accept things you cannot change, and focus on the present moment instead of worrying about the past or future.

Learning new ways to look at problems can also help. When faced with a challenge, try to see it as something you can handle or learn from, rather than a disaster. Practice positive self-talk by reminding yourself of your strengths and past successes.

Do things you enjoy and that give you a sense of purpose. Whether it is a hobby, a creative activity, volunteering, or spending time in nature, making time for what you love helps fill your life with meaning and joy.

Long-term stress management is not about avoiding all stress but about giving yourself the tools to recover and stay healthy. By making these strategies a part of your daily life, you can handle challenges with greater ease, bounce back from setbacks, and enjoy more peace and happiness every day.

The Role of Exercise and Diet

Exercise and diet play a huge role in how your body and mind handle stress. When you take care of your physical health, you give yourself a better chance to stay calm, focused, and positive, even when life gets busy or challenging.

Regular exercise is one of the best ways to manage stress. When you move your body — whether it is walking, running, dancing, cycling, or playing a sport — your brain releases chemicals called endorphins. These natural "feel-good" chemicals boost your mood and help your body relax. Exercise also burns off stress hormones, like adrenaline and cortisol, that build up when you are worried or tense. Even short bursts of movement, like stretching, taking the stairs, or a quick walk outside, can make you feel better right away.

Exercise also helps you sleep more deeply and feel more energetic during the day. When you are well-rested and full of energy, it is easier to handle whatever comes your way. It does not matter if you are not an athlete or do not have fancy equipment. The key is to find an activity you enjoy and try to move your body every day, even if it is just for a few minutes.

Diet is just as important when it comes to managing stress. The foods you eat affect your energy, mood, and ability to focus. Eating regular, balanced meals with plenty of fruits, vegetables, whole grains, and protein helps keep your blood sugar steady. This gives you consistent energy throughout the day and prevents mood swings or crashes. Drinking enough water is essential, too, as dehydration can make you feel tired and irritable.

Try to limit foods and drinks that can make stress worse. Too much caffeine from coffee, tea, or energy drinks can make you feel jittery or anxious. Sugary snacks and drinks can give you a quick burst of energy, but leave you feeling tired soon after. Highly processed foods, like chips and fast food, do not provide your body with the nutrients it needs to cope with stress.

Instead, choose whole foods that help your body function at its best. Foods rich in vitamins and minerals—like leafy greens, nuts, seeds, fish, eggs, beans, and yogurt—help support your brain and nervous system. Some people find it helpful to plan meals and snacks ahead of time so they are less likely to grab unhealthy options when they are busy or stressed.

Eating and exercising are not just about your physical health—they affect your mind and emotions too. When you make healthy choices, you feel stronger, more confident, and better able to manage life's challenges. Exercise and diet do not need to be perfect; just making a few small changes can make a big difference.

Taking care of your body through regular movement and nourishing foods, you give yourself a solid foundation for handling stress. Over time, these habits will help you feel more balanced, positive, and ready to enjoy all that life has to offer.

Mindfulness Practices for Stress Relief

Mindfulness is a simple but powerful practice that can help you manage stress and feel more peaceful every day. Being mindful means paying full attention to the present moment, noticing your thoughts and feelings without judging them, and bringing your mind back when it starts to wander. Mindfulness helps you slow down, calm your body, and respond to stress with greater patience and understanding.

One of the easiest ways to practice mindfulness is through mindful breathing. You do not need any special tools or a lot of time—just a quiet moment. Sit comfortably, close your eyes if you like, and focus on your breath. Notice how the air feels as you breathe in and out. If your mind drifts to worries or plans, gently bring your attention back to your breath. Even a few minutes of mindful breathing each day can make a big difference in how calm and clear you feel.

Another mindfulness practice is a body scan. This involves paying close attention to each part of your body, one area at a time. Lie down or sit comfortably, and start by noticing how your feet feel. Move slowly up your body — legs, hips, stomach, chest, arms, hands, neck, and head. As you focus on each part, notice any sensations, tension, or relaxation you feel. If you find any tightness, breathe into that area and imagine it softening. A body scan helps you relax your muscles and become more aware of where you hold stress.

Mindful walking is an excellent practice if you prefer movement. Take a slow walk, either indoors or outside, and pay close attention to each step. Notice how your feet touch the ground, how your legs move, and the rhythm of your breath. Listen to the sounds around you, feel the air on your skin, and watch the colors or shapes you see. Mindful walking turns a regular walk into a calming, stress-relieving activity.

You can also practice mindfulness in everyday activities. While eating, focus on the taste, texture, and smell of your food. When washing your hands, pay attention to the temperature of the water and the feeling of the soap. Even during chores like washing dishes or folding laundry, you can slow down, notice your movements, and bring your mind back to what you are doing.

Guided mindfulness meditations are widely available in books, apps, and online videos. These can help you get started and provide gentle reminders to stay present and kind to yourself. Some people also like to keep a mindfulness journal, writing down moments when they felt calm, grateful, or aware of their thoughts and feelings.

Practicing mindfulness regularly can lower stress, improve your focus, and help you feel more balanced. Over time, you may notice that you are less easily upset by challenges and more able to enjoy the good moments in your life. Mindfulness is not about stopping your thoughts or becoming someone else — it is about noticing, accepting, and caring for yourself, just as you are. By adding small moments of mindfulness to your day, you give yourself a simple, powerful tool for stress relief and a happier, healthier mind.

CHAPTER 11

Cultivating Self-Love

Self-love means treating yourself with kindness, respect, and understanding — no matter what is happening in your life. It is not about being perfect or never making mistakes. Instead, self-love is about accepting who you are, valuing your strengths, and caring for yourself the same way you would care for a good friend. In this chapter, you will learn why self-love matters, how it affects your confidence and happiness, and simple ways to nurture it every day. By cultivating self-love, you create a strong foundation for growth, healing, and a more joyful life.

Understanding Self-Love vs. Selfishness

Self-love is sometimes misunderstood. Some people think loving yourself means being selfish or caring only about your own needs. In truth, self-love is about showing yourself respect and kindness so that you can be your best for yourself and others. Self-love is healthy, honest, and caring — it helps you grow, heal, and face challenges with confidence.

When you practice self-love, you take time to look after your body, mind, and emotions. You listen to your own needs and give yourself permission to rest or say no when you need to. Self-love also means speaking kindly to yourself, forgiving your mistakes, and believing in your worth. These habits help you feel more balanced and less likely to feel burned out or overwhelmed.

Selfishness, on the other hand, is when someone thinks only of themselves and ignores or hurts the needs of others. A selfish person might take more than their fair share, refuse to help, or not listen to others' feelings. Selfishness can damage relationships, create distance, and make others feel unimportant. It often leads to loneliness, frustration, or guilt.

It is important to remember that self-love is not about putting yourself above everyone else. Instead, it is about caring for yourself so you can bring your best self to your relationships, work, and daily life. When you fill your cup, you have more energy and kindness to share with others.

Here is a simple table to help you understand the difference between self-love and selfishness:

Self-Love	Selfishness
Respects own needs and others' needs	Ignores others' needs
Sets healthy boundaries	Refuses to compromise
Practices kindness and self-care	Focuses only on personal gain
Shares and helps when possible	Takes without giving back
Forgives self and learns from mistakes	Blames others, avoids responsibility
Nurtures healthy relationships	Damages or ignores relationships
Feels balanced, joyful, and fulfilled	Often feels empty or unsatisfied

Practicing self-love means honoring your own needs while also respecting the needs and feelings of others. It helps you live with more balance, happiness, and confidence—making life better for you and for everyone around you.

Daily Practices for Self-Love

Building self-love is not something that happens overnight. It is a gentle process that grows stronger with small, caring actions each day. These daily practices help you show kindness and respect to yourself, making it easier to feel happy, balanced, and confident.

Start by speaking kindly to yourself. Notice your inner voice and the words you use when you think about yourself. If you catch yourself saying harsh or harmful things, pause and try to replace those words with gentle encouragement. Instead of "I can't do anything right," say, "I am learning and doing my best." Treat yourself with the same patience you would show a good friend.

Make time each day for self-care. This can be as simple as taking a few deep breaths, enjoying a healthy meal, going for a walk, or making sure you get enough sleep. Taking care of your body is a way to show yourself that you matter. Small self-care actions add up and send a powerful message to your mind and heart.

Practice gratitude by noticing things you appreciate about yourself and your life. Each day, write down one or two things you are grateful for, no matter how small. Maybe you finished a project, helped a friend, or made time to rest. Gratitude enables you to focus on what is good and reminds you of your strengths.

Set healthy boundaries with your time and energy. It is okay to say no to things that drain you or do not feel right. Permit yourself to rest, take breaks, or step back from relationships or activities that leave you feeling stressed or unappreciated. Boundaries are a form of self-respect and help you protect your well-being.

Celebrate your progress, no matter how small it may seem. Notice when you take a step forward, learn something new, or handle a challenge. Take a moment to feel proud of yourself. You do not need to wait for significant achievements—every bit of growth is worth celebrating.

Forgive yourself when you make mistakes. No one is perfect, and everyone has days when things go wrong. If you mess up or fall short of your expectations, be gentle with yourself. Learn from the experience, let go of guilt, and remind yourself that you are still worthy of love and respect.

Connect with supportive people who care about you. Spend time with friends, family, or groups that make you feel valued and understood. Let them know how you feel and allow yourself to receive their kindness. Positive relationships are a source of strength and can help you see the good in yourself.

Practicing these simple acts of self-love every day, you build a stronger, kinder relationship with yourself. Over time, self-love becomes a natural part of your life, helping you handle stress, face challenges, and enjoy life with a fuller, happier heart.

Healing from Past Hurts

Everyone experiences pain, disappointment, or rejection at some point in life. Sometimes, these hurts come from mistakes you have made. Other times, they come from the actions or words of others. Carrying past hurts can make it hard to move forward, feel confident, or trust again. But healing is possible, and you can take small steps each day to let go and feel lighter.

The first step to healing is allowing yourself to feel your emotions. It is normal to feel sad, angry, or even embarrassed about what happened. You do not have to pretend everything is okay. Permit yourself to sit with your feelings for a while—cry, write in a journal, talk to someone you trust, or spend some quiet time reflecting. Naming your feelings is the beginning of understanding them.

Sometimes, old hurts stick around because you replay them in your mind over and over. Try to notice when this happens and gently guide your thoughts back to the present. Mindfulness, or simply focusing on what is happening right now, can help you break the cycle of rumination.

Remind yourself that the past is over, and you have the power to shape your present and future.

Forgiveness can be a big part of healing, but it does not mean forgetting or saying what happened was okay. Forgiving yourself or others is about letting go of the hold that pain has on your life. You might say, "I am choosing to let this go for my peace." Sometimes, forgiveness is a process that takes time — be patient and kind with yourself as you work through it.

Focus on learning from the experience. Ask yourself, "What did I discover about myself or others?" You may find new strength, courage, or the ability to set better boundaries. Even painful experiences can teach valuable lessons that help you grow wiser and more compassionate.

Take care of yourself as you heal. Surround yourself with people who support and encourage you. Spend time doing things that bring you comfort or joy, like spending time in nature, listening to music, creating art, or practicing relaxation exercises. Self-care is not selfish — it is essential for rebuilding your sense of safety and self-worth.

If your past hurts feel too heavy to handle alone, consider talking to a counselor, therapist, or trusted mentor. Professional support can offer new perspectives, guidance, and tools for healing. You do not have to go through the process by yourself.

Healing from past hurts does not happen in a single day, but with patience, support, and self-compassion, the pain will fade. Over time, you will find more room in your heart for happiness, confidence, and hope. Remember, you deserve to heal and feel whole again. Each step you take, no matter how small, is a sign of strength and the beginning of a brighter future.

Building Healthy Boundaries

Setting healthy boundaries is a vital part of self-love and well-being. Boundaries are the invisible lines you draw to protect your time, energy, feelings, and personal space. They help you decide what is okay for you and what is not. When you have healthy boundaries, you can say yes to what feels right and no to what does not, without feeling guilty or afraid.

Healthy boundaries start with knowing your own needs and limits. Take time to notice how you feel in different situations. Do you feel tired after spending time with certain people? Do you need quiet time alone to recharge? Pay attention to signs that you are feeling stressed, overwhelmed, or taken for granted. These are clues that your boundaries may need to be stronger.

Learning to say no is an important skill. You do not have to agree to every request or invitation, even if you want to please others. If something does not feel right, it is okay to decline politely. You can say, "I am not able to help with that right now," or "Thank you for inviting me, but I need some time for myself." Saying no is not rude or selfish—it is a healthy way to take care of yourself.

Being transparent and honest about your boundaries is also essential. Let others know what you are comfortable with and what you are not. For example, if you need quiet time after work, tell your family or roommates, "I need some time alone when I get home." If someone speaks to you in a way that feels hurtful, you can say, "I do not like being spoken to that way." Clear communication helps others understand your needs and reduces confusion or resentment.

Respecting other people's boundaries is just as important as protecting your own. Listen when someone says no or tells you what they need. Healthy relationships are built on mutual respect and understanding.

It can be challenging to set boundaries, especially if you are not used to it or if people around you resist. Remember that setting boundaries is not about pushing people away. It is about creating a space where you feel safe, valued, and able to be your true self. When you respect your limits, you have more energy and kindness to share with others.

Sometimes, you may need to adjust your boundaries as life changes. What worked for you in the past might not work now, and that is okay. Be flexible and keep checking in with yourself about what you need.

If someone does not respect your boundaries, stand firm and repeat your needs calmly. If they continue to push, it may be necessary to spend less time with them or seek support from others.

Building healthy boundaries takes practice and patience, but it leads to greater confidence, healthier relationships, and a stronger sense of self. By honoring your needs and standing up for yourself, you create a life that feels safer, more peaceful, and full of respect, both for yourself and those around you.

Self-Love and Relationships

Self-love is not only crucial for your happiness, but it also plays a significant role in building healthy and lasting relationships with others. When you love and respect yourself, you are better able to give and receive love, set healthy boundaries, and choose relationships that are good for you.

When you practice self-love, you bring your best self into your relationships. You know your worth and do not rely on others to make you feel valued. This helps you avoid unhealthy patterns, like needing constant approval, feeling jealous, or giving up your needs to please someone else. You are able to share your true feelings, ask for what you need, and respect your partner's needs as well.

Loving yourself also means you are less likely to accept mistreatment or stay in toxic situations. If someone speaks to you unkindly, ignores your feelings, or tries to control you, your self-love gives you the strength to stand up for yourself or walk away if needed. You know that you deserve to be treated with kindness and respect.

In a healthy relationship, both people encourage each other to grow. When you feel confident and secure in yourself, you support your partner's dreams, celebrate their successes, and help them through challenges. You do not feel threatened by their growth because you know that your value does not depend on comparison or competition. This creates trust and deepens your connection.

Self-love also helps you positively handle conflicts. Instead of blaming yourself for every problem, you can look at challenges honestly and work together to find solutions. You are willing to apologize when you make mistakes and to forgive when your partner does. Self-love makes it easier to be patient, gentle, and understanding.

Taking care of yourself outside of your relationship is another way to bring more love into it. Spend time with friends, follow your interests, and make room for the things that bring you joy. This keeps your life balanced and helps you stay happy, even when things are difficult.

Sometimes, loving yourself means taking a break from relationships to focus on your healing and growth. It is okay to spend time alone, reflect on what you need, and build your self-worth before sharing your life with someone else.

Self-love is not about being perfect or never needing help. It is about accepting yourself fully, caring for your needs, and believing that you are worthy of love, both from yourself and others. When you start from a place of self-love, every relationship in your life can grow stronger, healthier, and more joyful.

CHAPTER 12

Practicing Gratitude

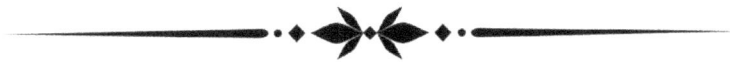

—··◆·◆··—

Gratitude is the simple act of noticing and appreciating the good things in your life. It might be as big as reaching a goal or as small as enjoying a cup of tea on a quiet morning. Practising gratitude helps you focus on what is working instead of what is missing or going wrong. In this chapter, you will learn why gratitude matters, how it can lift your mood and support your inner strength, and simple ways to make it a natural part of your day. By practising gratitude, you invite more joy, hope, and peace into your life, no matter what challenges you face.

The Power of Gratitude

Gratitude has the power to change the way you see your life and the world around you. When you practice gratitude, you shift your attention from problems and worries to the good things you already have. This simple habit can make your days brighter, your mood lighter, and your relationships stronger.

Gratitude helps you notice the positive moments you might otherwise miss — a smile from a friend, a warm meal, a sunny afternoon, or even just a few minutes of quiet. When you take time to appreciate these things, you realise that there is good in every day, no matter how small. This new way of seeing your life helps you feel more hopeful and less focused on what you do not have.

Research shows that people who regularly practice gratitude feel happier and less stressed. They are more optimistic and better able to cope with life's challenges. Gratitude can also improve your physical health, helping you sleep better, feel more energetic, and even boost your immune system. When you feel grateful, your body relaxes and your mind becomes more peaceful.

Gratitude also brings people closer together. When you express thanks to others, you build trust and connection. Saying "thank you" lets someone know you value them, and it can inspire kindness and support in return. Sharing gratitude with family, friends, or coworkers creates a positive circle where everyone feels appreciated.

Practicing gratitude can help you handle difficult times, too. When life feels challenging or overwhelming, looking for even the most minor good things can give you strength. It does not mean ignoring your problems, but it helps you see that challenges do not erase all the good in your life. Sometimes, just writing down one thing you are thankful for can help you feel a little lighter.

Gratitude is a skill you can build with practice. It starts with simply noticing what is going well in your life, then taking a moment to feel thankful. You can write your thoughts in a journal, share them with someone you care about, or pause and smile when something good happens.

The more you practice gratitude, the more natural it becomes. Over time, your mind gets used to looking for the good, and you find yourself feeling more positive and hopeful, even on tough days. Gratitude does not change the facts of your life, but it changes the way you experience them, turning ordinary moments into reasons to feel blessed.

Opening your heart to gratitude, you invite more happiness, peace, and connection into your life. It is a small habit with a significant impact, and it is available to you every single day.

Ways to Practice Gratitude

There are many simple ways to practice gratitude and make it a regular part of your daily life. You do not need special tools or a lot of extra time. With just a few minutes and a willing heart, you can start feeling the benefits of gratitude right away.

One easy way to practice gratitude is to keep a gratitude journal. Every day, write down one, two, or three things you are thankful for. They can be big, like getting a new job or hearing good news, or small, like enjoying your favourite food or a beautiful sunset. Writing these things down helps you focus on the good moments and remember them, especially on days when you need a little extra encouragement.

Another way to practice gratitude is to say thank you often. Express your thanks to the people around you, whether it's your family, friends, coworkers, or even strangers. You can thank someone for their help, their kindness, or just for being there. A simple thank you can brighten someone's day and make you feel good, too.

Take a few moments each day to pause and notice the positive things around you. You might sit quietly and think about what went well today, who made you smile, or what you enjoyed. This habit trains your mind to look for the good, even in the middle of a busy or stressful day.

Practicing gratitude can also be as simple as sharing your feelings with others. Tell a friend or loved one how much you appreciate them. You might write a note, send a message, or say it in person. When you share gratitude, it strengthens your relationships and spreads more kindness in the world.

You can practice gratitude by giving back. Do something thoughtful for someone else — hold the door, share a meal, offer a compliment, or help with a task. Acts of kindness remind you of the good in your life and help you feel more connected to others.

Some people like to use gratitude reminders throughout the day. You might put a note on your mirror, set a daily alarm, or keep a special object that reminds you to pause and be thankful. These gentle prompts can help you remember to look for the good, even on hard days.

Gratitude can also be part of your daily routines. Before bed, think of three things you are grateful for that happened during the day. When you wake up, set an intention to notice and appreciate the positive moments ahead. With time, these routines will help you see that there is always something to be thankful for.

Practicing gratitude in small, simple ways each day, you train your mind to focus on the positive. Over time, you will find yourself feeling happier, more hopeful, and more at peace, no matter what challenges you face. Gratitude is a powerful tool that can transform your life, one thankful thought at a time.

The Science behind Thankfulness

Thankfulness, or gratitude, is more than just a nice feeling — it changes your brain and body in ways that can make you happier and healthier. Scientists have studied gratitude and found that it has real, positive effects on your mood, relationships, and even your physical health.

When you feel thankful, your brain releases "feel-good" chemicals such as dopamine and serotonin. These chemicals help lift your mood and make you feel more relaxed and content. Practicing gratitude regularly can train your brain to look for positive things in your life, even during tough times. Over time, this habit can make you more optimistic and better able to handle stress.

Research has shown that people who practice thankfulness feel happier and more satisfied with their lives. They are less likely to feel anxious or depressed and tend to have more energy and better sleep. Grateful people also recover faster from setbacks and find it easier to focus on solutions instead of getting stuck on problems. By noticing and appreciating the good, you create a sense of hope that helps you bounce back when life gets hard.

Gratitude also helps your body. Studies have found that grateful people have stronger immune systems and lower blood pressure. They are less likely to get sick and often experience fewer aches and pains. This is because thankfulness can reduce the amount of stress in your body, which is known to weaken your health over time. When you practice gratitude, you help your body relax, heal, and protect itself.

Thankfulness has a significant impact on your relationships, too. When you express gratitude to the people around you, it builds trust, closeness, and respect. Saying thank you makes others feel valued and encourages more kindness in return. People who practice gratitude are often more patient, generous, and willing to forgive. This helps build stronger friendships, family bonds, and teamwork at work or in school.

The benefits of gratitude do not depend on your age, background, or where you live. Anyone can practice thankfulness and feel the difference. Even if life is challenging, noticing just one thing each day to be grateful for can help shift your perspective and bring a little more joy into your world.

Scientists agree that the more you practice gratitude, the easier it becomes to see the good around you. Your brain creates new pathways that make thankfulness a natural part of your thinking. This does not mean you will never feel sad or stressed, but it does mean you will be better equipped to handle those feelings and find hope even in difficult moments.

Thankfulness is a simple, powerful tool for building a happier, healthier life. By making gratitude a daily habit, you are not just changing your outlook—you are also changing your brain, your body, and your relationships for the better. The science is precise: practicing thankfulness works, and it is available to everyone, every single day.

Daily Gratitude Journaling

Daily gratitude journaling is one of the simplest and most effective ways to bring more thankfulness into your life. It is a habit anyone can start—no special skills or fancy notebooks required. All you need is a few minutes each day and a willingness to notice the good around you.

The idea behind gratitude journaling is to write down the things you are thankful for. You can do this at any time of day, but many people find it helpful to write in the morning to start their day on a positive note, or in the evening to reflect on the good things that happened. You can use a notebook, a journal app on your phone, or even a piece of scrap paper. The key is to make it a regular part of your routine.

Start by writing down three things you are grateful for each day. These can be big or small. Maybe you are thankful for a delicious meal, a call from a friend, a moment of laughter, or simply having a roof over your head. Try to be specific. Instead of writing "I'm grateful for my family," you might write, "I'm grateful that my sister listened to me today when I was feeling down." The more detailed you are, the more meaningful your gratitude practice becomes.

Do not worry if you repeat yourself sometimes—some blessings show up often, and that is perfectly fine. The important thing is to keep noticing and recording them. If you have a tough day, look for small things, like the comfort of a warm drink, a kind word, or a quiet moment. Even on the hardest days, there is always something to appreciate.

You can also use your gratitude journal to reflect on challenges. Ask yourself, "What lesson did I learn today?" or "What strength did I use to get through a hard moment?" This helps you see growth and progress, even in difficult times.

If you want, you can add drawings, photos, or little mementos that make you smile. There are no rules—your gratitude journal is for you, and it can be as creative or straightforward as you like.

Over time, gratitude journaling changes the way you see the world. You begin to notice more good things around you, and you train your mind to focus on hope instead of worry. When you look back through your journal, you will see how many positive moments have filled your days. This can give you extra comfort and encouragement when you need it most.

Gratitude journaling is a gift you give yourself each day. It brings more joy, calm, and balance to your life and helps you remember that even in difficult times, there is always something to be thankful for. By making this simple habit part of your routine, you can build a more positive and peaceful mindset, one grateful thought at a time.

Negativity with Gratitude

Everyone faces negative thoughts and tough days from time to time. It is natural to feel frustrated, sad, or worried when things do not go as planned. Sometimes, negativity can even become a habit—your mind may focus more on what is wrong than what is going well. The good news is that practicing gratitude is a powerful way to shift your focus and bring more light into your life, even during challenging moments.

Gratitude helps you notice the good, no matter how small, and reminds you that there is always something to appreciate. When you feel yourself getting stuck in negative thinking, pause and take a deep breath. Ask yourself, "Is there something I can be thankful for right now?" It could be as simple as a comfortable chair, a kind smile, or a memory that makes you laugh.

Try to challenge negative thoughts by looking for positives in the same situation. If you are frustrated about a long wait, you may have extra time to listen to your favorite music or practice patience. If you feel disappointed by a setback, remind yourself of past times when you overcame challenges or learned something new. Gratitude does not ignore your problems—it gives you the strength to face them with hope and resilience.

Writing your feelings in a gratitude journal is a great way to break the cycle of negativity. When you write down things you are thankful for, your mind starts searching for more good around you. Even on difficult days, finding just one small thing to appreciate can help lift your mood and change your perspective. Over time, this practice can make positive thinking feel more natural and automatic.

Another helpful way to use gratitude is by reaching out to others. When you thank someone for their help or kindness, you strengthen your connection and create a joyous moment for both of you. Complimenting a friend, sharing your appreciation, or simply saying thank you can help you feel more hopeful and less alone.

Mindfulness can also play a role in overcoming negativity. Take a few minutes to sit quietly and notice your breath, your senses, or the sounds around you. Let go of worries about the past or future, and focus on the present. In this moment, try to name one thing that brings you comfort or peace.

Practicing gratitude does not mean you have to ignore your struggles or pretend that everything is perfect. Life has ups and downs, and it is okay to feel negative emotions sometimes. The key is to remember that your challenges do not erase all the good in your life. By making gratitude a regular habit, you give yourself the tools to rise above negativity, bounce back from setbacks, and see life through a brighter, more hopeful lens.

With time and practice, you will find that gratitude can soften the hardest days and help you find light, even when things feel dark. This simple shift in focus can bring more peace, joy, and strength into your everyday life—one grateful thought at a time.

CHAPTER 13

Nurturing Relationships

Healthy relationships are one of the most significant sources of happiness and support in life. Whether with family, friends, a partner, or even coworkers, caring connections help you feel understood, valued, and less alone. Nurturing relationships is not about grand gestures—it is about showing up, listening, and building trust over time. In this chapter, you will learn why strong relationships matter, what makes them grow, and practical ways to create deeper, more meaningful bonds with the people in your life. By investing in your relationships, you make every day richer and more fulfilling.

Why Relationships Matter

Relationships are at the heart of a happy and meaningful life. Whether it's with family, friends, a partner, or people in your community, the connections you make shape your experiences, influence your health, and give you a sense of belonging. Even if you are someone who enjoys time alone, having supportive relationships is still important—they remind you that you are cared for, understood, and never truly alone.

One of the main reasons relationships matter is that they provide emotional support during life's ups and downs. When you have someone to share your worries and joys with, it becomes easier to handle stress, bounce back from setbacks, and celebrate successes. Just knowing that someone will listen to you when you need to talk, offer advice, or give a hug can make even the hardest days feel lighter. Emotional support is not just about solving problems; it's also about knowing someone is on your side no matter what.

Relationships also play a significant role in your physical health. Studies show that people who have strong, positive connections tend to live longer and enjoy better health overall. Supportive relationships can lower stress, boost your immune system, and even reduce your risk of heart disease. When you feel connected and cared for, your body responds in healthy ways—your sleep improves, your energy increases, and you're more likely to make positive choices like eating well and exercising.

Having good relationships helps you grow as a person. Being close to others teaches you essential skills like empathy, patience, forgiveness, and how to solve problems together. You learn to see the world through someone else's eyes, to understand different perspectives, and to appreciate what makes each person unique. Relationships challenge you to be honest, kind, and responsible—not just for yourself, but for the people you care about.

Another reason relationships matter is that they give life meaning and purpose. When you share your life with others, you create memories, celebrate traditions, and build a history together. You feel needed and valued, not just for what you do but for who you are. Helping others, supporting friends through tough times, or raising a family all bring a sense of fulfillment that goes beyond personal achievements. Relationships remind you that you are part of something bigger than yourself.

Strong relationships also help you navigate changes and challenges. Life is full of unexpected twists, like moving to a new place, changing jobs, or losing a loved one. During these times, the support and encouragement of friends and family can make transitions smoother and less overwhelming. You can lean on others for strength, share your feelings, and know that you are not facing difficulties alone.

Relationships matter because they shape your happiness. The people you spend time with influence your mood, your outlook, and even your habits. Positive, supportive relationships lift you, inspire you to do your best, and help you see the bright side of life. They are a source of laughter, joy, and comfort. On the other hand, unhealthy or harmful relationships can leave you feeling drained, anxious, or lonely. That's why it's essential to surround yourself with people who bring out the best in you and who appreciate you for who you are.

Building and keeping good relationships takes effort, but the rewards are worth it. Little things—like listening, sharing, showing gratitude, and spending quality time together—help strengthen your bonds. Honest conversations, acts of kindness, and supporting each other's dreams all contribute to deeper, more meaningful connections. Even when disagreements happen, working through them respectfully helps build trust and understanding.

Relationships are also where you practice self-love and set healthy boundaries. When you know your own needs and communicate them clearly, your relationships become more balanced and respectful. You learn that it's okay to say no, to ask for what you need, and to take care of yourself while caring for others. Healthy boundaries allow both people to feel safe and valued, making the relationship stronger and more enjoyable for everyone.

In today's fast-paced world, it can be easy to let relationships slip down the list of priorities. Work, technology, and busy schedules sometimes get in the way. But making time for the people who matter most is one of the best investments you can make in your well-being and happiness. Whether it's a phone call, a text, a shared meal, or a walk together, small moments of connection add up and keep relationships strong.

Relationships matter because they connect you to the heart of what it means to be human. They bring comfort during hard times, joy in the good times, and a sense of belonging all the time. By caring for your relationships and showing up for the people you love, you not only enrich your own life but also help create a kinder, more caring world for everyone.

Building Strong, Healthy Connections

Building strong, healthy connections with others is one of the most rewarding parts of life. Good relationships do not just happen by chance—they are created through kindness, trust, respect, and steady effort. No matter your age or background, you can build lasting bonds with friends, family, a partner, or anyone you meet by practicing a few simple but powerful habits.

The foundation of any healthy connection is trust. Trust means you feel safe to share your thoughts and feelings, knowing that the other person will listen, keep your confidence, and treat you with care. To build trust, start by being honest and open. Share your true feelings and let others know what matters to you. Honesty can feel a little scary at first, especially if you are worried about being judged. But the more you practice it, the stronger your relationships will become. When you are honest, you encourage others to be honest, too.

Respect is just as important as trust. In strong relationships, both people respect each other's opinions, choices, and boundaries. Respect shows up in how you talk to each other, how you listen, and how you handle disagreements. You can show respect by listening carefully, waiting your turn to speak, and accepting that the other person might see things differently from you. Even when you disagree, respect allows you to talk things through calmly and reasonably.

Good communication is the lifeblood of healthy connections. This means not just talking, but also listening with your full attention. When someone speaks, try to really hear what they are saying, instead of planning your reply. Ask questions, repeat back what you heard, or say, "Tell me more." Listening shows you care and want to understand, which makes others feel valued and close to you.

Another essential part of building strong relationships is showing appreciation. Let people know what you love or admire about them. Say thank you for their help, support, or simply for being themselves. Small gestures of appreciation—a note, a text, a smile, or a compliment—go a long way toward keeping relationships warm and positive. When you focus on what is good in others, you invite more kindness into your life as well.

Quality time together is also key. Life gets busy, but making time to connect is worth it. Try to set aside moments, even if short, where you can be fully present with the people you care about.

99

Share a meal, take a walk, play a game, or sit and chat. Turn off your phone and give your attention to the person in front of you. These moments help deepen your bond and create happy memories you will treasure.

Healthy connections also require boundaries. Boundaries are limits you set to protect your well-being and respect the well-being of others. They help you say yes to what feels good and no to what does not. You should set boundaries around your time, energy, or personal space. Clear, kind communication about your boundaries makes relationships stronger and more honest. It is okay to take breaks, ask for what you need, or say no when something is not right for you.

Handling disagreements and challenges together is another way to build strong connections. No relationship is perfect—there will always be bumps along the way. When problems come up, try to work as a team instead of blaming or criticizing. Talk openly about what is wrong, listen to each other's feelings, and look for solutions together. Apologize when you make a mistake, and be willing to forgive when someone else does. Every time you work through a conflict, you build more trust and understanding.

Support each other's growth and dreams. Encourage your friends and loved ones to follow their passions, learn new things, and reach their goals. Celebrate their achievements and stand by them during tough times. When you cheer for someone else's success, you strengthen your relationship and build a culture of support that benefits everyone.

Building strong, healthy connections is not about being perfect or doing everything right. It is about showing up, caring, and trying your best. It is also about taking care of yourself, so you have the energy and love to share with others. When you nurture your well-being, you bring your best self to your relationships.

Be patient. Great relationships grow over time, through shared experiences, trust, and a willingness to work through challenges together. Every step you take to listen, show respect, express appreciation, and spend quality time is an investment in a happier, more connected life.

Practicing these habits, you create relationships that lift you up, help you grow, and fill your days with meaning and joy. Building strong, healthy connections is one of the best gifts you can give yourself and the people around you.

Navigating Conflict with Grace

Conflict is a natural part of every relationship. No matter how close you are to someone, there will be times when you disagree, misunderstand each other, or want different things. Navigating conflict with grace is not about avoiding disagreements or pretending everything is perfect—it is about handling challenging moments with honesty, respect, and a willingness to listen and grow.

The first step to managing conflict is to stay calm. When emotions are high, it is easy to say things you do not mean or to get defensive. If you notice yourself getting upset, take a few deep breaths, count to ten, or ask for a short break before continuing the conversation. Giving yourself a moment to calm down helps you think more clearly and speak more kindly.

Start the conversation by focusing on your feelings, not blaming the other person. Use "I" statements to share your experience. For example, say, "I feel hurt when plans change at the last minute," instead of, "You never stick to plans." This approach keeps the discussion centered on your feelings and avoids making the other person feel attacked.

Listening is just as essential as speaking. Give the other person a chance to share their side without interrupting or judging. Show you are listening by nodding, making eye contact, or repeating back what you heard. Sometimes, all someone needs is to feel heard and understood before they can move forward.

Try to understand where the other person is coming from. Ask questions if you are not sure what they mean, and be open to the idea that their perspective might be different from yours. Remember, it is possible to disagree and still respect each other. Looking for common ground — something you both agree on — can help shift the conversation from conflict to cooperation.

It is also helpful to stay focused on the issue at hand, rather than bringing up old problems or unrelated complaints. Stick to the current situation, and do your best to avoid words like "always" or "never," which can make things feel more dramatic than they are. If the conversation starts to go off track, gently steer it back to what matters most right now.

Sometimes, you might not reach complete agreement, and that is okay. The goal of conflict resolution is not to "win" but to find a way forward that works for both people. Look for solutions that meet everyone's needs as much as possible. This might mean compromising or trying something new. Be willing to let go of being right if it means keeping the relationship strong.

Apologizing can be a powerful part of navigating conflict with grace. If you realize you made a mistake, said something hurtful, or misunderstood, say you are sorry. A genuine apology helps rebuild trust and shows that you care about the other person's feelings. Forgiving the other person, when you are ready, is just as important. Holding onto anger or resentment can keep you stuck, while forgiveness makes space for healing and growth.

Setting healthy boundaries during conflict is also essential. If a conversation becomes too heated or if you feel disrespected, it is okay to pause and suggest continuing later. Respect your limits and let the other person know what you need to feel safe and heard. Boundaries help keep conflict constructive instead of harmful.

After a conflict, take time to care for yourself and the relationship. Check in with the other person and talk about what you learned from the experience. Celebrate the progress you made, even if things are not perfect. Over time, working through conflicts together builds more trust, understanding, and resilience in your relationship.

It is normal to feel nervous or uncomfortable during disagreements, but facing conflict with grace gets easier with practice. Each time you handle a tough moment with patience and respect, you grow stronger and more confident in your ability to solve problems and maintain healthy connections.

No relationship is free from conflict, and that is not a sign of failure. It is an opportunity to learn, grow, and become closer. When you meet conflict with an open heart and a calm mind, you can turn even the most challenging conversations into moments of understanding and connection.

Navigating conflict with grace is a skill that will serve you well in every part of life. It helps you build relationships that are honest, strong, and able to weather any storm. By staying calm, listening deeply, and looking for solutions, you make every relationship more resilient and loving, one conversation at a time.

Communication in Relationships

Communication is the backbone of every healthy relationship. It is how you share your feelings, thoughts, needs, and dreams with the people who matter most. Whether you are talking with a partner, family member, or friend, transparent and honest communication helps build trust, prevent misunderstandings, and deepen your connection over time. Good communication is not just about the words you use — it is also about listening, understanding, and respecting each other's point of view.

In any relationship, open and honest conversation is key. This means being willing to talk about both the good and the difficult things. Share what makes you happy, what worries you, and what you hope for the future. When you are honest about your feelings, you make it easier for the other person to understand you and support you in the ways you need. Holding back or keeping secrets can lead to confusion, hurt feelings, and distance over time.

Active listening is just as essential as speaking. When someone you care about is sharing, please give them your full attention. Put away distractions like phones or TV, make eye contact, and show that you are listening by nodding or giving small verbal responses like "I see" or "That makes sense." Don't interrupt or jump in with your own story right away — let them finish what they want to say. If you are not sure what they mean, ask gentle questions or repeat what you heard in your own words to check for understanding.

Tone of voice and body language matter a lot in communication. Sometimes, what you say and how you say it send different messages. If your words are caring but your voice sounds sharp or your arms are crossed, the other person may feel confused or hurt. Try to keep your voice calm and your posture open, even when talking about tough topics. A gentle touch, a smile, or a relaxed posture can all make conversations feel safer and more positive.

It's essential to make time for honest conversations, especially when life gets busy. Set aside regular times to talk, whether over a meal, during a walk, or before bed. Regular check-ins help keep you connected and let minor issues be solved before they turn into big problems. When you know you have time to talk, you are less likely to bottle up feelings or let misunderstandings grow.

Don't be afraid to talk about your needs and boundaries. It's healthy to let others know what you are comfortable with, what you need help with, or when you need space. You can say things like, "I need some quiet time after work," or "It helps me when you check in during the day." Sharing your needs is not selfish—it is a way to take care of yourself and help the relationship thrive.

Conflict is a natural part of relationships, and how you communicate during disagreements makes a big difference. Try to focus on the issue, not the person. Use "I" statements instead of blaming, such as "I feel upset when plans change suddenly," instead of "You always change things at the last minute." Be willing to listen to the other side and look for solutions together. Remember, it's okay to take a break if things get too heated—sometimes a little space helps both people calm down and come back ready to solve the problem.

Gratitude and appreciation are also essential parts of communication. Make it a habit to thank the people in your life, compliment their strengths, and show that you notice the good things they do. Small acts of appreciation—like saying thank you, leaving a kind note, or giving a hug—can lift someone's spirits and make your bond stronger.

Communication is not about being perfect or always agreeing. It's about showing up, being real, and working through things together. It's okay if you make mistakes or have awkward moments—what matters is your willingness to try, learn, and keep the conversation going.

Sometimes, you may need support to improve communication, especially if you are dealing with old patterns or difficult emotions. Talking with a counselor, reading books, or attending workshops together can offer new skills and help you grow closer.

The more you practice open and honest communication, the easier it becomes. Over time, you will find that your relationships feel safer, more loving, and more resilient, able to face any challenge life brings. Communication is the bridge that keeps you connected, turning ordinary moments into chances for understanding, laughter, and love. By making it a priority, you create relationships that are strong, joyful, and built to last.

Supporting Others While Supporting Yourself

Being there for others is one of the most rewarding parts of any relationship. Whether you are comforting a friend, helping a family member through a hard time, or encouraging a partner, offering support can strengthen your bond and bring you closer. But supporting others is not just about giving—it is also essential to care for your well-being so you can help from a place of strength, not exhaustion. Balancing support for others while supporting yourself is a skill that brings more joy, resilience, and harmony into your life.

When someone you care about is going through a tough time, you might feel a strong urge to help in any way you can. This is a sign of your kindness and empathy. Sometimes, you can lend a hand with practical help, like running errands or offering advice. Other times, just listening with patience and an open heart can mean the world to someone who is struggling. Often, the most incredible comfort you can offer is simply being present and showing you care.

Listening deeply is one of the best ways to support others. Please give them your full attention, set aside distractions, and allow them to share their feelings at their own pace. You do not have to fix everything or have all the answers—just being there, nodding, and saying things like "That sounds really hard," or "I'm here for you," is often enough. Try not to interrupt or judge, and remember that sometimes people need to express their feelings before they are ready to look for solutions.

It is also essential to respect your limits. While it feels good to help, you can only give what you have. If you are tired, stressed, or dealing with your challenges, it is okay to take a step back and care for yourself first. You might say, "I want to be here for you, but I need a little time to recharge. Can we talk later?" This does not mean you are selfish—it means you value your well-being, which helps you show up as your best self when you are ready.

Supporting others should not come at the cost of your own health, happiness, or personal boundaries. If you notice yourself feeling overwhelmed, resentful, or exhausted, it may be time to pause and reflect on what you need. Make sure you are getting enough rest, enjoying your hobbies, and spending time with people who uplift you. When you care for yourself, you have more patience, energy, and love to give.

Another key part of supporting others is knowing when to ask for help. If someone's needs are more than you can handle, or if you feel out of your depth, encourage them to reach out to a professional or another trusted person. Saying, "I think you might benefit from talking to a counselor," or "Would you like me to help you find more support?" shows that you care deeply and want the best for them.

You are not responsible for solving everyone's problems. Sometimes, all you can do is listen, offer comfort, and remind your loved one that they are not alone. Trying to take on too much can lead to burnout or even harm the relationship if you start to feel resentful or overwhelmed. Supporting others is most helpful when it comes from a place of balance.

Setting healthy boundaries is a loving act for both yourself and the other person. Boundaries help you stay clear about what you can and cannot offer, which protects your energy and helps avoid misunderstandings. For example, you could limit long phone calls late at night, or say no to taking on extra responsibilities when you are already busy. Boundaries are not walls—they are gentle guides that help keep relationships strong and positive.

Taking care of yourself is not selfish. It is essential if you want to be there for others in the long run. Self-care might mean taking quiet time to rest, practicing mindfulness, going for a walk, or connecting with friends who support you. When you recharge your energy and fill your cup, you bring more compassion and understanding to every relationship.

Celebrate the moments of connection and support you share with others. Helping someone through a hard time is a gift, and so is allowing others to help you when you need it. By caring for both yourself and those around you, you create a circle of support that lifts everyone higher.

Balancing support for others while caring for yourself is a journey, not a one-time task. It is about listening, setting boundaries, and making space for both giving and receiving. With practice, you will find that you can support others with a generous heart while also honoring your own needs, building relationships that are strong, loving, and healthy for everyone involved.

CHAPTER 14

Mindfulness and Meditation for Inner Strength

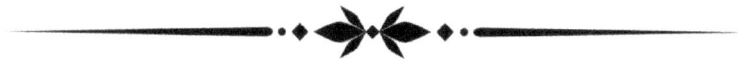

—◆◆◆—

Mindfulness and meditation are powerful tools for building inner strength and creating a sense of calm in everyday life. These practices help you focus on the present moment, reduce stress, and become more aware of your thoughts and feelings without judgment. In this chapter, you will learn how mindfulness and meditation can support your emotional well-being, make you more resilient, and bring more peace and clarity to your life. With a few simple steps, you can use these gentle practices to feel stronger, more balanced, and better able to handle whatever comes your way.

What Is Mindfulness?

Mindfulness is the practice of paying attention to the present moment, on purpose, and without judgment. It means noticing what is happening inside you — your thoughts, feelings, and body sensations — as well as what is happening around you. When you are mindful, you are fully awake to the here and now, rather than worrying about the past or the future.

At its core, mindfulness is about awareness. Most of the time, our minds are busy jumping from one thought to another. We might replay old conversations, worry about what could go wrong, or plan what we need to do next. Mindfulness gently invites us to slow down and focus on what is happening right now. It does not mean you have to clear your mind or ignore your thoughts. Instead, it means watching your thoughts come and go without getting caught up in them.

For example, practice mindfulness while eating a meal. Rather than eating quickly or being distracted by your phone or TV, you focus on the taste, smell, and texture of each bite. You notice how the food feels in your mouth, how your body feels as you eat, and the simple act of breathing in and out. If your mind wanders, you gently bring your attention back to your meal.

Mindfulness can also help you notice your emotions. If you feel stressed, anxious, or upset, mindfulness encourages you to pause and observe your feelings. You might think, "I notice I'm feeling nervous," without judging yourself for it or trying to push the feeling away. This creates space between you and your emotions, which can help you respond with more calm and kindness.

One of the best things about mindfulness is that anyone can practice it, anytime and anywhere. You do not need special skills or equipment. You can be mindful while walking, showering, listening to music, or even washing dishes. The key is to bring your full attention to whatever you are doing and to notice your experience with curiosity and acceptance.

Practicing mindfulness regularly can help you feel more grounded and less overwhelmed by life's ups and downs. It can lower your stress, improve your mood, and help you make clearer choices. Over time, mindfulness can even change the way your brain responds to stress, making you more resilient and at ease.

Mindfulness is not about being perfect or always feeling peaceful. It is about coming back to the present moment, again and again, with patience and kindness. By making mindfulness a part of your daily life, you build a strong foundation for inner strength, emotional balance, and lasting well-being.

Meditation Techniques for Beginners

Meditation is a simple and gentle practice that anyone can learn. It helps you quiet your mind, relax your body, and become more aware of your thoughts and feelings. You do not need any special equipment or experience—just a few minutes a day and a willingness to try. Here are some easy meditation techniques that are perfect for beginners:

1. Mindful Breathing

Sit comfortably with your back straight and your hands resting in your lap or on your knees. Close your eyes if you feel comfortable. Focus your attention on your breath. Notice how the air feels as it moves in and out of your nose or mouth. Try to keep your attention on each inhale and exhale. If your mind starts to wander, gently bring it back to your breath. You can do this for just two or three minutes at first and slowly increase the time as you get used to it.

2. Body Scan Meditation

Lie down or sit in a comfortable position. Close your eyes and take a few slow, deep breaths. Starting with your toes, bring your attention to each part of your body in turn—your feet, legs, hips, stomach, chest, arms, hands, neck, and head. Notice any tension, warmth, or relaxation in each area. If you find a spot that feels tight or sore, breathe into it and let it relax. The body scan helps you connect with your body and release stress.

3. Guided Meditation

Many people find it helpful to use a recorded meditation or an app with gentle instructions. Guided meditations walk you through each step and often include calming music or nature sounds. You can find free guided meditations online or in many smartphone apps. These are great for beginners who want some support while they learn.

4. Loving-Kindness Meditation

This meditation focuses on sending kind thoughts to yourself and others. Sit quietly, breathe slowly, and repeat a simple phrase in your mind, such as, "May I be happy. May I be healthy. May I be safe?" Then, think of someone you love and repeat the same wish for them. Gradually, extend your kind wishes to friends, acquaintances, and even people you have difficulties with. Loving-kindness meditation helps increase compassion and understanding.

5. Walking Meditation

If you find it hard to sit still, try walking meditation. Stroll and focus on the sensation of your feet touching the ground, your breath, and the movement of your body. Notice the sights, sounds, and smells around you as you walk. Walking meditation can be done indoors or outdoors and is a great way to practice mindfulness in motion.

You do not need to do all these meditations at once. Choose one that feels comfortable and try it for a few minutes each day. If your mind wanders or you feel restless, that is entirely normal — bring your focus back without judging yourself. With practice, meditation can become a peaceful part of your routine, helping you feel calmer, clearer, and more centered every day.

Using Mindfulness to Overcome Anxiety

Anxiety is a feeling of worry, nervousness, or unease that can make daily life feel overwhelming. Everyone feels anxious at times, but when anxiety becomes intense or frequent, it can be hard to focus, relax, or enjoy life. Mindfulness is a gentle and effective tool that can help you manage anxiety by bringing your attention back to the present moment and calming your mind.

When you practice mindfulness, you learn to notice your anxious thoughts and feelings without judging them or trying to push them away. Instead of getting lost in worries about the future or regrets about the past, you gently bring your attention to what is happening right now. This simple shift helps you realize that, in this moment, you are safe and okay.

One of the easiest ways to use mindfulness for anxiety is mindful breathing. When you feel anxious, your breath often becomes shallow and quick. Take a few moments to slow down and focus on each inhale and exhale. Breathe in slowly through your nose, hold for a second, then breathe out gently through your mouth. Notice how your chest and belly rise and fall. Even just a few mindful breaths can help relax your body and calm your thoughts.

Another helpful technique is grounding. Anxiety can make your mind race with worries, but grounding exercises help bring your focus back to the present. Try the "5-4-3-2-1" method: Notice five things you can see, four things you can touch, three things you can hear, two things you can smell, and one thing you can taste. This exercise helps interrupt anxious thinking and reminds you of your surroundings right now.

Mindfulness also teaches you to observe your thoughts rather than react to them. When you notice a worrying thought, pause and say to yourself, "That is just a thought, not a fact." Let the thought pass by like a cloud in the sky. By watching your thoughts come and go, you begin to see that you do not have to believe or act on every worry your mind creates.

You can also use mindfulness in daily activities to help reduce anxiety. Try being fully present while washing your hands, eating a meal, or going for a walk. Notice the sights, sounds, smells, and sensations as they happen. Bringing your attention to simple tasks gives your mind a break from worry and helps you feel more grounded.

Mindfulness is a skill that takes practice. You might not feel calm right away, and that is okay. The important thing is to keep coming back to the present moment, again and again, with patience and kindness toward yourself.

Using mindfulness to overcome anxiety does not mean you will never feel anxious again. It means you will have a gentle tool to help you handle anxious moments, calm your body, and find peace even when life feels uncertain. Over time, mindfulness can help you feel stronger, more balanced, and more in control of your thoughts and feelings.

Mindful Self-Reflection Practices

Mindful self-reflection is the practice of looking inward with kindness and curiosity, rather than judgment or criticism. It helps you understand your thoughts, feelings, actions, and habits so you can learn, grow, and make positive changes. By combining mindfulness with self-reflection, you become more aware of who you are and what you truly need.

A straightforward practice is mindful journaling. Find a quiet space and set aside a few minutes each day to write about your experiences, thoughts, and emotions. The goal is not to judge or "fix" anything, but to notice and describe what is happening inside you. You might start with questions like, "How am I feeling right now?" or "What thoughts keep coming up for me?" Writing down your reflections helps you process your feelings and see patterns over time.

Another way to practice mindful self-reflection is through guided meditation. Sit comfortably, close your eyes, and focus on your breath. As you settle, gently bring a question into your mind, such as, "What do I need most today?" or "What am I grateful for?" Let your thoughts and feelings arise naturally, without pushing or forcing answers. Notice what comes up and return to your breath if your mind gets busy. After a few minutes, you can write down any insights or sit with what you discovered.

Body scan meditations can also be a form of self-reflection. As you move your attention through different parts of your body, notice where you feel tension, comfort, or energy. Ask yourself, "What is my body trying to tell me?" or "How does my body feel when I think about certain situations?" Listening to your body's signals helps you care for yourself in more profound ways.

Mindful self-reflection can also happen in everyday activities. Take a moment during your day—perhaps while walking or waiting in line—to check in with yourself. Notice your emotions, your posture, and your thoughts. Are you feeling stressed, relaxed, or excited? What might be causing those feelings? This gentle awareness helps you respond to life with intention rather than automatic reaction.

It is essential to approach self-reflection with self-compassion. Be gentle with yourself, especially if you notice difficult emotions or patterns you want to change. Remind yourself that everyone has strengths and struggles, and that self-reflection is a tool for growth, not for self-blame.

Over time, mindful self-reflection helps you better understand your values, triggers, dreams, and needs. It becomes easier to make choices that match who you are and what you want for your life. You become more patient, resilient, and kind to yourself and to others.

Making mindful self-reflection a regular practice supports your journey toward inner strength, peace, and personal growth. By looking inward with awareness and care, you lay the foundation for lasting change and a more profound sense of well-being.

Integrating Mindfulness into Daily Life

Mindfulness does not have to be limited to meditation or quiet moments—it can become a natural and supportive part of your everyday life. When you integrate mindfulness into your daily routine, you learn to slow down, pay attention, and respond to situations with greater calm and clarity, no matter where you are or what you are doing.

Start your day with a few mindful breaths. As soon as you wake up, take a moment to notice your breathing. Feel the air moving in and out, and let yourself become aware of how your body feels. This gentle practice sets a peaceful tone for the day and helps you begin with intention.

Mindful eating is another simple way to bring awareness into your daily life. Instead of rushing through meals or eating while distracted, try to focus on the taste, smell, and texture of your food. Chew slowly, notice the colors on your plate, and appreciate each bite. Mindful eating not only makes meals more enjoyable but also helps you listen to your body's hunger and fullness signals.

Bring mindfulness to your commute, whether you are walking, driving, or using public transport. Pay attention to the sights, sounds, and sensations around you. Notice the feeling of your feet on the ground, the rhythm of your breath, or the way sunlight hits your skin. If you find your mind wandering to worries or plans, gently return your attention to the present moment.

You can practice mindfulness while doing chores. Washing dishes, folding laundry, or tidying your space can become opportunities for awareness. Focus on the sensations—the warmth of the water, the smell of soap, the movement of your hands. Let go of rushing and be present with the task.

Mindful pauses throughout the day can help you reset and refocus. Take a few slow, deep breaths before starting a new task, making a decision, or entering a meeting. These brief moments give your mind a break and help you respond rather than react, especially during stressful times.

At work or school, give your full attention to one task at a time. Multitasking can make you feel scattered and stressed. By focusing on a single activity, you become more effective and less overwhelmed.

Practice mindful listening in your relationships. When someone is speaking, please give them your full attention without interrupting or thinking about what you'll say next. Notice their words, body language, and tone. Mindful listening builds trust, reduces misunderstandings, and deepens your connection with others.

Your day with gratitude. Before going to sleep, think of one or two things that went well or brought you joy. This helps your mind settle and supports a restful night.

Integrating mindfulness into daily life is about being present, one moment at a time. You do not need to be perfect or mindful all day long—even small efforts make a difference. With practice, mindfulness becomes a natural habit, helping you handle challenges with patience, enjoy simple pleasures, and live each day with more awareness and peace.

Advanced Meditation Methods

Once you are comfortable with basic meditation techniques like mindful breathing, body scans, and guided sessions, you should explore advanced meditation methods. These practices can help deepen your awareness, increase your sense of calm, and build even greater inner strength.

While advanced meditations take time and patience, anyone can learn them with practice and an open mind.

1. Visualization Meditation

Visualization meditation involves creating positive images or mental "movies" in your mind to inspire peace, motivation, or healing. Sit quietly and picture a calm place, like a beach, forest, or mountain. Imagine all the details—the sounds, colors, and scents. You can also visualize yourself achieving a goal, feeling healthy, or facing challenges with confidence. Visualization can help reduce anxiety, boost confidence, and support healing.

2. Mantra Meditation

A mantra is a word or phrase that you repeat quietly to yourself during meditation. Common mantras include words like "peace," "calm," or "let go." In traditional practices, people might use Sanskrit phrases, such as "Om." Choose a mantra that feels meaningful to you. Sit comfortably, close your eyes, and repeat the mantra softly, either aloud or silently. Focusing on the sound and rhythm of your mantra can help quiet your mind and bring you deeper into meditation.

3. Mindful Movement (Yoga, Tai Chi, Qigong)

Mindful movement practices combine gentle exercise with focused awareness. Yoga, Tai Chi, and Qigong are all examples. These activities use slow, flowing movements and conscious breathing to help you connect with your body and the present moment. Practicing mindful movement can reduce stress, increase flexibility, and improve your overall sense of balance and energy.

4. Chakra Meditation

Chakra meditation comes from ancient Indian traditions. It involves focusing your attention on different "energy centers" in your body, known as chakras. As you meditate, imagine energy flowing through these centers—from the base of your spine up to the top of your head. You might visualize each chakra as a spinning wheel of light, each with its color. Chakra meditation is believed to help balance your emotions, boost vitality, and promote healing.

5. Loving-Kindness (Metta) Meditation

This advanced method builds on the basic loving-kindness practice. In Metta meditation, you systematically send kind wishes to yourself, then to loved ones, acquaintances, people you have difficulty with, and finally to all beings everywhere. The repetition of kind phrases expands your sense of compassion and connection.

6. Silent Retreats

For those who want to take meditation even deeper, silent retreats offer an extended period of focused practice. These retreats, which can last from a day to several weeks, often involve periods of sitting and walking meditation, mindful eating, and complete silence. While challenging, retreats can help you experience profound calm and clarity.

Advanced meditation methods are not about being perfect or reaching a certain level. They are opportunities to explore your mind and heart with curiosity and patience. With regular practice, these techniques can lead to more profound peace, resilience, and self-discovery, enriching your journey to inner strength and well-being.

CHAPTER 15

Visualization and Mental Rehearsal

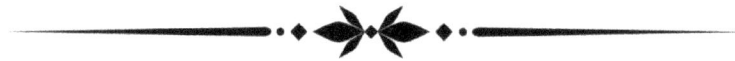

———————•·◆◆◆·•———————

Visualization and mental rehearsal are potent tools for building inner strength, boosting confidence, and reaching your goals. These practices involve using your imagination to create positive pictures and experiences in your mind before they happen in real life. By seeing yourself succeed, handling challenges, or staying calm under pressure, you train both your mind and body for success. In this chapter, you will discover how visualization and mental rehearsal work, why they are effective, and how to use them in your everyday life to unlock your full potential and create the outcomes you want.

The Science behind Visualization

Visualization is more than just daydreaming. It is a mental exercise that uses your imagination to create detailed pictures of what you want to achieve or experience. Scientists have discovered that visualization can change the way your brain and body respond, helping you prepare for challenges, improve your skills, and build confidence.

The power of visualization starts in your brain. When you imagine yourself doing something — whether it is giving a speech, playing a sport, or facing a tricky situation — your brain "rehearses" the activity as if it is happening. Brain scans show that the same parts of your brain are activated during visualization as when you perform the task. This means that visualizing yourself succeeding can help build the neural pathways and muscle memory you need to perform better in real life.

Athletes have used visualization for decades to improve their performance. Before a big race, for example, runners often picture themselves crossing the finish line strong and confident. They imagine each step, each breath, and the feeling of accomplishment at the end. This mental practice helps prepare both their minds and bodies for the real event, increasing their chances of success. The same strategy is used by musicians, public speakers, and even surgeons — anyone who wants to perform at their best.

Visualization works because your brain does not always know the difference between a real event and a vividly imagined one. When you create detailed mental images, your body responds as if you are experiencing the event. Your heart rate might go up, your muscles may tense, and you can even feel a rush of excitement or calm, depending on what you imagine. Over time, these physical responses become more familiar, so you are less likely to feel nervous or unsure when the real moment comes.

Another reason visualization is effective is that it helps you set clear goals and stay motivated. When you regularly picture yourself achieving your dreams, you are more likely to believe in your ability to make them happen. This positive mindset encourages you to take action, keep trying after setbacks, and stay focused on your goals. Visualization also helps you notice opportunities and solutions that you might miss if you are only focused on your fears or doubts.

Researchers have found that visualization can also reduce stress and anxiety. By imagining yourself calm and in control during challenging situations, you teach your brain and body to respond with relaxation instead of panic. This can make a big difference in situations like job interviews, exams, or public speaking, where nerves might otherwise get in the way.

Visualization is not about pretending that life will always be perfect or that challenges will disappear. Instead, it is about preparing yourself to handle whatever comes with confidence, focus, and resilience. You can use visualization to practice facing fears, overcoming obstacles, or even healing from past hurts.

To make visualization work for you, practice regularly. The more you use your imagination in a focused, intentional way, the stronger the effects will be. With time, you will find that you feel more prepared, positive, and ready to reach your goals.

The science behind visualization is precise: by creating detailed mental images of success, you train your brain and body to work together, building the skills and confidence you need to turn your dreams into reality. Visualization is a simple but powerful tool that can help you grow, overcome challenges, and live your best life.

Guided Visualization Techniques

Guided visualization is a practical and enjoyable way to use your imagination to support your goals, reduce stress, and build confidence. You do not need special skills or experience—just a quiet place, a few minutes, and a willingness to try. With guided visualization, you follow along with gentle instructions, either from a recording, a book, or your inner voice, as you create calming or motivating images in your mind.

One simple technique is the "Safe Place Visualization." Close your eyes, take a few slow breaths, and picture a place where you feel completely safe and at ease. This could be a real location—a favorite spot in nature, a cozy room, or the beach — or it could be an imaginary space filled with soothing colors and light. Notice all the details: What do you see, hear, and feel? Imagine the temperature, the sounds, and even the scents around you. Let yourself fully relax in this safe space, knowing you can return to it anytime you feel stressed or anxious.

Another powerful technique is "Future Self Visualization." In this exercise, you imagine yourself in the future, having already achieved a goal or overcome a challenge. Close your eyes and picture what you look like, how you stand, and what expression is on your face. Notice how you feel — proud, calm, joyful, or firm. What are you doing? Who is around you? Imagine hearing someone congratulate you or feeling a sense of relief. Please spend a few minutes enjoying this future success, letting it fill you with motivation and hope.

For those looking to boost confidence before a specific event — like a speech, interview, or exam — the "Mental Rehearsal" technique is beneficial. Picture yourself preparing for the event, walking into the room, and taking a deep breath. Imagine yourself speaking, answering questions with confidence, or completing each step with focus. If your mind drifts to worries, gently bring it back to a positive, successful outcome. Notice how your body feels — relaxed, steady, and capable. This rehearsal helps train both your mind and body to respond with calm and skill when the real moment arrives.

The "Healing Visualization" technique is perfect for times when you are feeling hurt or needing extra comfort. Close your eyes, relax your body, and picture a gentle, warm light surrounding you. Imagine this light moving through your body, bringing healing, comfort, and peace to any area that feels tense, tired, or painful. You might even picture your worries floating away or being transformed into strength. Healing visualizations can be especially helpful at bedtime or when you need to nurture yourself.

Guided visualization can be done with the help of recordings, apps, or even just your voice. Many people find it helpful to listen to a calm guide who gently describes each step and prompts you to imagine different sensations or scenes. You can find free guided visualizations online, in meditation apps, or through therapists and coaches.

If you prefer to guide yourself, write down a short script or speak quietly to yourself as you move through each step. Start by relaxing your body, then bring your attention to your breath. As you describe the scene in your mind, use all your senses — see, hear, feel, and even smell or taste what is around you. The more detail you add, the more real and powerful the visualization becomes.

Guided visualization regularly, even for just five or ten minutes a day, can help you feel calmer, more hopeful, and more confident in reaching your goals. Remember, your imagination is a powerful tool. With a bit of practice, you can use it to relax, heal, and set yourself up for success in all areas of life.

Using Visualization for Confidence and Resilience

Visualization is not just about imagining success—it is also a powerful way to build absolute confidence and resilience that you can use in everyday life. When you see yourself handling challenges, speaking up, or bouncing back from setbacks in your mind, you give your brain and body a "preview" of what it feels like to be confident and strong. Over time, this practice can help you face real situations with more calm, courage, and determination.

To use visualization for confidence, start by thinking about a situation where you want to feel more self-assured. It could be a presentation at work, meeting new people, taking a test, or simply speaking your truth. Find a quiet place to sit comfortably, close your eyes, and take a few deep breaths to relax. Now, picture yourself in that situation—see every detail as clearly as you can. Imagine yourself standing tall, speaking clearly, and feeling calm and steady inside.

As you move through the scene in your mind, notice how your body feels. Imagine your heart beating calmly, your breathing slow and deep, and a sense of quiet strength in your chest and shoulders. Hear your voice sounding strong and sure. Picture others listening, nodding, or smiling. Allow yourself to feel proud of how you are handling things. If doubts or worries pop up, gently let them float by, and return your focus to the positive outcome you are creating.

Repeat this practice often, especially before moments that make you nervous. Each time you visualize yourself succeeding, you strengthen the pathways in your brain that support confidence. Over time, these mental "rehearsals" will help your real-life actions feel more natural and less scary.

Visualization can also build resilience, which is your ability to recover from setbacks and keep going, even when things get tough. To practice, choose a past situation where you faced a challenge, or imagine a future obstacle. See yourself meeting the challenge with patience and resourcefulness. In your mind, watch yourself take a deep breath, look for solutions, ask for help if needed, and stay kind to yourself along the way.

Now imagine the moment you bounce back—maybe you find a new way forward, learn something valuable, or get up and try again. Feel the sense of relief and pride that comes with not giving up. Let this feeling of resilience settle in your mind and body.

You can also use visualization to prepare for unexpected stress or setbacks. Picture yourself encountering a problem, feeling anxious or disappointed, and then reminding yourself that you have the strength to cope. Imagine using calming techniques—like deep breathing or positive self-talk—and see yourself regaining your balance. Visualize yourself moving through the tough moment and coming out stronger on the other side.

The key to making visualization work for confidence and resilience is regular practice and as much detail as possible. Use all your senses, and truly feel the emotions of success and recovery. Even if you do not believe it at first, trust that your brain is learning from each session.

With time, visualization becomes a quiet source of strength you can draw on whenever you need it. By imagining yourself handling life's ups and downs with confidence and resilience, you prepare your mind and body to do the same in reality. This simple, powerful tool can help you move through challenges, try new things, and bounce back from setbacks with more hope, courage, and self-belief.

Overcoming Limiting Beliefs with Mental Rehearsal

Limiting beliefs are thoughts or ideas you hold about yourself that keep you from reaching your full potential. They might sound like "I am not good enough," "I always fail at this," or "People like me do not succeed." These beliefs are often picked up from past experiences, criticism, or even the stories we hear from others. Over time, they can become so automatic that you start to believe them without question. But the good news is, you can change limiting beliefs—and mental rehearsal is a powerful way to do it.

Mental rehearsal is like practicing for success in your mind. Instead of replaying negative thoughts or past failures, you choose to imagine yourself acting with confidence, courage, and strength. This new "mental movie" helps your brain get used to new, positive possibilities.

To begin, identify a limiting belief that often holds you back. Maybe it is something like "I am too shy to speak up," or "I never finish what I start." Please write it down, and notice when it comes up in your daily life. The next step is to challenge that belief with a new, positive statement—called an empowering belief. For example, change "I am too shy to speak up" to "I can express my ideas with clarity," or "I never finish what I start" to "I am capable of following through."

Now, use mental rehearsal to practice this new belief. Find a quiet place to sit comfortably, close your eyes, and take a few deep breaths to relax. Picture a situation where your limiting belief usually appears. It could be a meeting, a social event, or starting a new project. Instead of seeing yourself struggle or stay silent, imagine yourself doing the opposite. See yourself speaking up, sharing your ideas, finishing your project, or stepping confidently into the situation.

Make the scene in your mind as vivid as possible. Notice how you look, stand, and move. Hear the sound of your voice—calm, steady, and clear. Feel the sense of accomplishment or relief as you do the thing you once thought you could not do. Picture other people responding positively, nodding, or showing support.

If doubts or negative thoughts show up while you are rehearsing, that is normal. Instead of fighting them, let them pass like clouds in the sky and gently bring your attention back to your empowering belief and positive actions.

118

Repeat this mental rehearsal often, daily if you can. The more you practice, the more your brain starts to accept this new belief as possible and actual. Over time, you may find yourself acting differently in real life, trying new things, and feeling more confident. Each small success reinforces your new belief, making it stronger and more natural.

It can also help to write your new empowering belief somewhere you will see it every day — on your mirror, in your journal, or on your phone. Say it out loud to yourself, especially when you notice the old belief creeping in.

Changing limiting beliefs is a journey, not something that happens overnight. But with patience and regular mental rehearsal, you can rewrite the stories you tell yourself and unlock abilities and courage you did not know you had. By imagining your success and practicing new ways of thinking, you open the door to growth, happiness, and a future full of new possibilities.

Case Studies: Athletes and High-Performers

Many of the world's top athletes, performers, and leaders use visualization and mental rehearsal as part of their daily routines. Their stories show how powerful these techniques can be — not just for winning medals or awards, but for building confidence, staying focused, and overcoming challenges.

One well-known example is Olympic swimmer Michael Phelps. Long before he jumped into the pool, Phelps would spend time every day visualizing his races. He pictured every stroke, every turn, and even imagined how he would react if something went wrong, like his goggles filling with water. During the 2008 Beijing Olympics, this practice paid off. In one race, his goggles did fill with water, and he could barely see, but because he had mentally rehearsed the situation so many times, he stayed calm and completed the race by counting his strokes. He won the gold medal, proving how powerful visualization can be when facing unexpected problems.

Another example comes from Serena Williams, one of the greatest tennis players in history. Williams often talks about the importance of mental imagery in her training. Before a big match, she spends quiet time visualizing herself serving, moving across the court, and handling tough points. She imagines feeling confident and strong, especially in high-pressure moments. This mental rehearsal helps her stay focused, keep her nerves in check, and perform at her best even under intense pressure.

Top basketball players, like LeBron James, also use visualization as part of their routine. LeBron is known for his strong mental game. He not only practices on the court but also spends time picturing himself making key shots, staying calm during big games, and leading his team. He credits visualization with helping him build the confidence and mental strength needed to play at the highest level.

Visualization is not limited to sports. Musicians, public speakers, and business leaders use these techniques to prepare for essential performances and meetings. World-class violinist Itzhak Perlman has spoken about mentally rehearsing every piece of music before stepping onto the stage. He imagines how each note will sound and how he will move his fingers, which helps him feel more prepared and confident when it is time to perform.

Even astronauts, who face extreme pressure and risk, use mental rehearsal before space missions. They imagine each step of their tasks, including possible emergencies, so that their brains and bodies are ready for anything. This kind of preparation is crucial when every action counts and mistakes can be costly.

What all these high performers have in common is a commitment to practicing not just their physical skills, but their mental skills as well. By taking the time to visualize success, overcome setbacks, and imagine themselves handling stress, they build inner strength that gives them an edge in competition and life.

You do not have to be an Olympic athlete or a famous performer to benefit from visualization and mental rehearsal. Anyone can use these tools to prepare for job interviews, school exams, public speaking, or significant life changes. By picturing yourself succeeding, handling setbacks, and staying calm, you train your mind and body to respond with confidence and resilience.

These real-world stories show that visualization is more than a simple exercise — it is a powerful tool that helps people of all backgrounds reach their highest potential, face challenges with courage, and achieve their dreams.

CHAPTER 16

Habit Engineering for Lasting Change

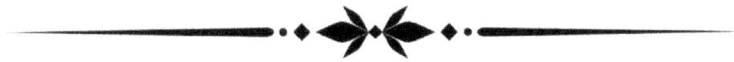

———··◆·◆··———

Creating lasting change in life often starts with small, daily habits. The way you think, act, and respond shapes your success, well-being, and inner strength over time. Habit engineering is about understanding how habits work and how you can design or reshape them to support your goals. In this chapter, you will discover how to build positive routines, break free from old patterns, and make changes that last. By learning the science and simple steps behind habit engineering, you can turn your dreams into reality, one small step at a time.

The Psychology of Habit Formation

Habits are the small actions and routines you repeat every day, often without even thinking about them. They shape your life, influence your success, and play a massive role in your happiness and well-being. Understanding the psychology behind how habits form can help you build new, positive routines and break free from old patterns that no longer serve you.

Habits are your brain's way of saving energy. Instead of having to make a new decision every time you brush your teeth, tie your shoes, or start your morning routine, your brain creates shortcuts—automatic behaviors that require little thought. These shortcuts are called "habit loops." Every habit loop has three main parts: the cue, the routine, and the reward.

The **cue** is the trigger that tells your brain to start a habit. It could be a specific time of day, a feeling, or something in your environment. For example, feeling stressed might be a cue to reach for a snack, or hearing your morning alarm might be a cue to start your coffee maker.

The **routine** is the action you take in response to the cue. This can be anything from brushing your teeth to scrolling through your phone or going for a run. Over time, routines become automatic—your brain does them without much conscious thought.

The **reward** is the benefit you get from the routine. Rewards can be physical (like a burst of energy from exercise), emotional (a sense of comfort from eating a favorite food), or social (praise from others for a job well done). The reward tells your brain that the habit is worth repeating, so the loop continues.

Your brain is wired to look for patterns. When it notices that a particular cue leads to a rewarding routine, it strengthens the connection, making the habit easier to repeat. This is why habits can be so hard to break—your brain has learned to expect the reward.

To change a habit, it helps to keep the same cue and reward but change the routine in between. For example, if stress is your cue and comfort is your reward, try replacing a routine of eating junk food with something healthier, like taking a walk or practicing deep breathing. Over time, your brain will start to connect the cue with the new routine and reward.

Habits also grow stronger with repetition. The more you practice a behavior, the more automatic it becomes. This is why it's essential to start small and focus on consistency. Even tiny changes, like drinking a glass of water each morning or writing down one thing you're grateful for, can add up to significant results when done regularly.

Motivation plays a role in habit formation, but it isn't always reliable. Some days you'll feel inspired, and other days you won't. The secret is to make your habits as easy and automatic as possible, so you stick with them even when motivation fades.

Environment matters, too. By changing your surroundings, you can make good habits easier and bad habits harder. For example, keeping healthy snacks visible and junk food out of sight, or setting out your workout clothes the night before, makes it easier to stick with new routines.

Understanding the psychology of habit formation gives you the power to design your habits, rather than letting them control you. With patience, consistency, and a little creativity, you can build positive routines that support your goals and well-being for the long term.

Identifying Keystone Habits

Some habits have a special power to create positive change in many areas of your life. These are called "keystone habits." A keystone habit is a small routine or behavior that, when practiced regularly, sets off a chain reaction of other good habits. Focusing on keystone habits can help you make significant improvements with less effort, because they naturally encourage other positive actions.

Identifying your keystone habits starts with paying attention to the routines that make you feel healthier, happier, or more productive. Think about the times in your life when things were going well. What daily actions or routines helped you stay on track? For many people, these habits include things like exercising, eating breakfast, keeping a journal, or going to bed at the same time each night.

One classic example of a keystone habit is regular physical activity. When you make exercise a part of your routine, you might notice that you sleep better, eat healthier, and feel more motivated throughout the day. Exercise not only benefits your body but can also boost your mood and give you more energy to handle challenges. As you start to feel better, you may naturally want to make other healthy choices, like drinking more water or cooking at home.

Another powerful keystone habit is planning your day. Taking just a few minutes in the morning or the night before to write down your goals, appointments, and priorities can help you feel more organized and in control. This small step often leads to better time management, less stress, and a greater sense of accomplishment as you check off your tasks.

Getting enough sleep is also a keystone habit for many people. When you go to bed and wake up at consistent times, your body and mind have a chance to rest and recharge. Good sleep improves your focus, mood, and even your immune system. It's much easier to stick to other healthy routines—like eating well or staying active—when you are well-rested.

Gratitude journaling is another example. Writing down a few things you are grateful for each day can shift your mindset, making you more optimistic and resilient. This practice often leads to noticing more good in your life, treating yourself and others with kindness, and handling stress more gracefully.

To identify your keystone habits, start by asking yourself a few questions:

- Which daily actions make me feel my best?
- What habits help me stay positive and motivated?
- Are there routines that set the tone for the rest of my day?
- When I feel off track, which habits am I missing?

Once you spot a keystone habit, make it a priority. Please keep it simple and easy to repeat. For example, if drinking water first thing in the morning helps you feel more awake and ready for the day, make it part of your morning routine. If a short walk after dinner lifts your mood, schedule it like a necessary appointment.

Remember, you do not need to change everything at once. Focusing on one keystone habit can start a ripple effect, making it easier to add more positive changes over time. As you build these foundation habits, you will find that creating a healthy, happy, and successful life feels much more natural and achievable.

Keystone habits are the building blocks of lasting change. By identifying and nurturing them, you give yourself the best chance to grow stronger, achieve your goals, and enjoy more balance every day.

The Role of Environment in Habit Building

Your environment has a powerful influence on your habits, often more than willpower or motivation alone. The spaces you live and work in, the people you spend time with, and the tools and cues around you can make it much easier—or much more complicated—to stick to new routines. Understanding and shaping your environment is one of the most innovative ways to support habit change and build a life that feels more balanced and positive.

Every habit begins with a cue, and many cues come from your surroundings. For example, if you keep a bowl of fresh fruit on your kitchen counter, you are more likely to reach for a healthy snack. If your workout clothes are laid out and ready in the morning, it becomes easier to exercise without extra effort. On the other hand, if your space is full of distractions or temptations—like snacks on your desk, a TV in your bedroom, or social media notifications—you might find yourself slipping back into old habits.

To build better habits, try to make good choices easy and convenient. Rearrange your environment so that healthy or productive actions are the most apparent option. For example, place your water bottle on your desk to remind you to drink, keep books within reach to encourage reading, or set up your workspace so you are comfortable and focused.

Removing barriers is just as important. If you want to watch less TV, put the remote out of sight or unplug the device. If you're going to eat less junk food, keep treats in a hard-to-reach cupboard or don't bring them home at all. Making bad habits less convenient reduces the chances you'll fall back into them, especially when you're tired or distracted.

Your digital environment matters, too. If you're trying to cut down on screen time or social media, log out of apps, turn off notifications, or move distracting icons off your home screen. Use technology to help you—set reminders for new habits, track your progress, or use calming apps to encourage mindfulness or sleep.

The people around you are a massive part of your environment. Spend time with those who support your goals and make healthy choices themselves. If your friends or family encourage you to stick with positive routines, you'll find it much easier to stay on track. Sometimes, joining a group or community with similar goals—like a walking club, book group, or online forum—can give you extra motivation and accountability.

Lighting, sound, and organization also play a role. A tidy, well-lit space makes it easier to focus and feel energized. Soft lighting and calming music can help you relax and sleep better at night. Even small changes, like adding plants or clearing clutter, can make your environment more welcoming and supportive of the habits you want to build.

Don't feel you need to change everything at once. Start with one or two simple adjustments that make your chosen habit easier to do. Over time, small changes to your environment will add up and help new routines feel more natural.

Habits are not just about self-control—they're about setting yourself up for success. By shaping your environment to support your goals, you reduce the friction and stress of making changes. You'll find it easier to stick to new habits, enjoy positive routines, and create a life that genuinely supports your health, happiness, and inner strength.

Breaking Bad Habits and Reinforcing Good Ones

Everyone has habits they wish they could change—whether it's biting their nails, procrastinating, eating too much junk food, or spending too much time on their phone. Breaking bad habits and building new, positive ones can feel challenging, but it is possible with patience, the right strategies, and a supportive environment.

The first step in breaking a bad habit is to notice when, where, and why it happens. Most bad habits have triggers—feelings, places, people, or times of day that make you more likely to act on them. For example, you might reach for snacks when you feel stressed or check your phone whenever you're bored. Keeping a simple habit journal for a week or two can help you spot patterns and understand what cues lead to your unwanted behaviors.

Once you know your triggers, try to interrupt the habit loop. This means breaking the link between the cue and your usual routine. If you tend to eat sweets when you're stressed, pause and ask yourself what you need. A short walk, a few deep breaths, or a glass of water could help instead. If you check your phone out of boredom, try keeping a book or puzzle nearby so you have a healthier way to pass the time.

Replacing a bad habit with a positive one is usually more effective than just trying to stop the behavior. The brain likes routines and rewards, so swapping an old habit for a new, healthy action makes the transition easier. For instance, instead of smoking when you feel anxious, try chewing gum or squeezing a stress ball. Over time, your brain will start to link the trigger with your new routine and reward.

Celebrate small wins. Breaking a habit takes time, and there will be days when you slip back into old patterns. Instead of getting discouraged, notice your progress and give yourself credit for every step forward. Positive reinforcement, like giving yourself a small treat, sharing your success with a friend, or marking your achievements on a calendar, helps strengthen good habits and keeps you motivated.

Accountability can also help. Tell someone you trust about the habit you're working to change, or join a group with similar goals. Support from others, even just a quick check-in, can boost your motivation and make you feel less alone in your journey.

Your environment plays a significant role in both breaking bad habits and reinforcing good ones. Remove temptations from your home or workspace, and set up reminders and cues for your new habits. If you want to drink more water, keep a bottle on your desk. If you want to read more, put your book in a visible spot. Making good habits easy and convenient while making bad habits less accessible increases your chances of success.

Be patient and kind to yourself. Changing habits takes time and practice. It's normal to have setbacks or tough days. What matters most is your willingness to try again and keep moving forward. Each effort, no matter how small, is a step toward lasting change.

Understanding your triggers, swapping in positive routines, and creating a supportive environment, you can break bad habits and build new ones that support your health, happiness, and goals. With steady effort, your good habits will become a natural and rewarding part of your everyday life.

Creating an Accountability System

Building new habits or changing old ones is much easier when you have support. An accountability system is simply a way to check your progress, stay motivated, and get encouragement when things get tough. It helps you keep your promises to yourself and makes your goals feel more real and achievable.

One of the simplest forms of accountability is sharing your goal with someone you trust. Tell a friend, family member, or coworker what you are working on—maybe it's walking every day, reading before bed, or eating healthier meals. Explain why the goal matters to you, and ask if they can check in with you regularly. Even just knowing that someone else cares about your progress can make a big difference in your commitment.

Some people like to find an "accountability partner"—someone with a similar goal who also wants support. You can motivate each other, celebrate successes, and help each other get back on track if you have a setback. For example, you might text each other each day after your workout, share healthy recipes, or talk about challenges you're facing. The partnership becomes a safe space for encouragement and honesty.

Joining a group is another powerful accountability tool. Look for clubs, classes, or online communities that focus on your area of growth. Whether it's a running group, a book club, or a support forum for breaking bad habits, being part of a group can inspire you to keep going, especially on hard days. The sense of belonging and friendly competition in a group setting often helps you stick with your new habits longer.

Self-accountability is essential, too. Keeping a habit tracker or journal gives you a clear picture of your progress. Use a calendar, an app, or a simple notebook. Each day, mark whether you completed your habit or not. Looking back and seeing your streak can boost your confidence and remind you of how far you've come. If you miss a day, don't get discouraged—focus on getting back on track the next day.

Rewards can be a significant part of your accountability system. Set small milestones and celebrate them. For example, after a week of sticking to your new bedtime, treat yourself to a favorite snack, a relaxing activity, or something special you enjoy. Rewards help reinforce good habits and make the process more enjoyable.

Setting up reminders is another helpful tool. Use alarms, sticky notes, or digital notifications to prompt you at key times. For example, a reminder on your phone to stretch every hour, or a sticky note on your bathroom mirror to start your day with gratitude. Reminders keep your new habit top of mind, especially when life gets busy.

If you find yourself struggling, don't be afraid to ask for help. Talk to your accountability partner or group about the obstacles you're facing. Sometimes just saying your struggles out loud makes them easier to manage, and you might get practical tips or encouragement you hadn't thought of.

Most importantly, be honest with yourself. Accountability is not about being perfect or never making mistakes. It's about noticing what works, learning from setbacks, and gently returning to your goals with fresh motivation. Celebrate every bit of progress, and remember that small steps forward are still steps in the right direction.

Creating an accountability system—whether with a partner, a group, or through self-tracking—you give yourself extra support, motivation, and the best chance for lasting success. With accountability, your habits become stronger, your goals become clearer, and your confidence in yourself grows with every step you take.

CHAPTER 17

Advanced Self-Reflection and Journaling Techniques

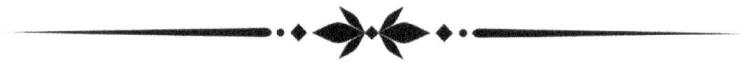

Self-reflection and journaling are powerful tools for personal growth and inner strength. As you continue your journey, you may find yourself ready to go deeper, exploring your thoughts, emotions, and experiences in new ways. Advanced self-reflection and journaling techniques help you uncover hidden patterns, gain fresh insights, and set meaningful intentions for your future. In this chapter, you will discover creative methods and thoughtful prompts that make your self-discovery process richer and more rewarding, supporting you as you grow and thrive.

Structured Journaling for Growth

Structured journaling is a focused way to use writing as a tool for personal growth. Instead of simply recording your thoughts or daily events, structured journaling uses specific prompts, formats, or routines to help you reflect more deeply and move forward with clear intentions. This kind of journaling can help you see patterns in your life, understand your emotions, and set meaningful goals.

One popular approach is the "question and answer" method. Each day, begin with a set of reflective questions, such as "What am I feeling right now?", "What went well today?", "What was challenging?", or "What can I learn from this experience?" By answering these questions honestly, you become more aware of your thoughts, feelings, and behaviors. Over time, this regular self-check builds greater self-awareness and emotional intelligence.

Another helpful format is the "goal and progress" journal. In this style, you start each week or month by writing down your key goals or intentions. Each day or every few days, you record what steps you took toward those goals, what worked, what didn't, and how you felt about your progress. This approach keeps you accountable and helps you celebrate small wins, while also giving you a space to problem-solve when you hit roadblocks.

The "gratitude and growth" journal combines appreciation with self-improvement. Begin each entry with a few things you are grateful for—big or small. Then, reflect on an area of growth or a challenge you are working through. Write about what you learned, what you could do differently, or how you want to approach things next time. This routine helps shift your mindset to focus on both the positive and the possibilities for change.

Using structured prompts is also a great way to spark new insights. Some prompts you might try include:

- "Describe a time you overcame fear—what helped you?"
- "What habits or beliefs would you like to change, and why?"
- "How have you grown in the past year?"
- "Who inspires you, and what qualities do you admire in them?"

You can use the same set of prompts for a week, a month, or whenever you need direction in your journaling practice. The regularity and structure keep your writing purposeful and help you dig deeper than surface-level thoughts.

To get the most from structured journaling, try to write at the same time each day or week. Find a quiet, comfortable place, and allow yourself to write freely, without judging your words. Remember, your journal is for you alone, so honesty and openness are key.

Structured journaling for growth is not about being perfect or always having the correct answers. It is about making space to listen to yourself, set intentions, and learn from your journey. Over time, these practices help you become more resilient, self-aware, and ready to face life's challenges with clarity and confidence.

Prompts for Deep Self-Discovery

Prompts for profound self-discovery are questions or statements that invite you to explore who you are on a deeper level. These prompts go beyond everyday worries or routines, helping you reflect on your values, dreams, fears, and the experiences that have shaped you. Using them in your journaling or quiet reflection can lead to powerful insights and positive change.

Here are some prompts to guide your self-discovery journey:

What are three moments in your life that changed you?

Think back to experiences—good or bad—that left a lasting mark. What did you learn from them? How did they shape your beliefs, behaviors, or goals?

When do you feel most alive, energized, or "yourself"?

Describe situations or activities that light you up. What do these moments have in common? How can you create more of them in your life?

What are your biggest fears, and where do they come from?

Explore what scares you most—not just on the surface, but deep down. How have these fears influenced your choices? What might help you face or understand them?

If you could give your younger self one piece of advice, what would it be?

Reflect on what you've learned since childhood or adolescence. What wisdom or comfort do you wish you'd had back then? How can you give that kindness to yourself now?

Who inspires you, and why?

Think about people you admire—family, friends, public figures, or even fictional characters. What qualities draw you to them? Are those qualities you'd like to strengthen in yourself?

What does your "ideal day" look like?

Imagine a day when everything goes right and you feel your best. What are you doing, who are you with, and how do you think? What steps could bring you closer to living that day for real?

What are you holding onto that no longer serves you?

Consider beliefs, habits, or relationships that may be weighing you down. Why is it hard to let go? What might life feel like if you released them?

When have you felt truly proud of yourself?

Describe a time you achieved something essential or acted with courage. How did that experience affect your confidence and self-worth?

What do you most want to create, change, or experience in the future?

Dream big—without limits. What calls to your heart? What steps could you take, even small ones, to move in that direction?

What does self-love mean to you right now?

How do you show care for yourself? Where do you struggle? What would make you feel more accepted and valued, just as you are?

Use one or two of these prompts each time you journal, or return to your favorites as you grow and change. Allow yourself to write honestly, without worrying about grammar or "right answers." If emotions come up, pause and give yourself compassion.

Profound self-discovery is a gentle journey, not a race. Each time you reflect on these prompts, you learn more about who you are, what matters most, and how you can live a life that feels true and fulfilling.

Using Reflection to Overcome Setbacks

Everyone faces setbacks and disappointments at some point in life. Whether it's a missed goal, a failed project, a broken relationship, or an unexpected challenge, setbacks can leave you feeling discouraged and unsure of how to move forward. However, reflection—taking time to look back, understand, and learn from what happened—can turn these challenging moments into powerful opportunities for growth.

The first step in using reflection to overcome setbacks is to allow yourself to feel whatever emotions arise. It's normal to feel sad, frustrated, or even angry when things don't go as planned. Give yourself space to process these feelings, whether through writing, talking to someone you trust, or simply sitting quietly with your thoughts. Ignoring your emotions or pretending nothing is wrong only makes it harder to heal.

Once you've given yourself some time, gently begin to reflect on what happened. Ask yourself: What exactly went wrong? What was in my control, and what wasn't? Sometimes, setbacks are the result of circumstances you couldn't change. Other times, there may be actions or choices you would make differently in the future. Try to look at the situation honestly but without blame or harsh self-criticism.

Next, look for lessons. What did this setback teach you about yourself, your goals, or your habits? You may have learned that you need more support, better planning, or a different approach. Every disappointment holds the seed of growth—sometimes, it reveals strengths you didn't know you had, like resilience, creativity, or the courage to try again.

Use your reflection to brainstorm new strategies. If you failed an exam, you may need a new study method or more rest. If a relationship ended, what can you learn about communication or setting healthy boundaries? Reflection turns regret into a plan for positive change.

It can help to write about your setback and what you're learning. Ask yourself:

- What would I do differently next time?
- What qualities helped me get through this moment?
- Who can I reach out to for support or advice?

Be sure to celebrate your efforts, even if the outcome wasn't what you hoped for. It takes courage to try, to care, and to dream big. Recognizing your effort reminds you that setbacks are part of growth, not signs of failure.

Use your reflection to set a small, positive action you can take next. It could be reaching out for help, making a new plan, or simply giving yourself more kindness. Taking even one step forward shows that you're willing to keep going, no matter what.

Setbacks are not the end of your story. With reflection, they become stepping stones to greater understanding, resilience, and future success. By looking back with honesty and compassion, you open the door to learning, healing, and new beginnings.

The Power of Daily Review

A daily review is a simple yet powerful habit that can help you grow, stay focused, and make steady progress toward your goals. By taking a few moments each day to look back, notice what went well, and consider what could be improved, you create a cycle of learning and growth that builds confidence and resilience over time.

The daily review does not have to be complicated or take a lot of time. At the end of each day, find a quiet spot, take a few deep breaths, and reflect on the past 24 hours. Ask yourself: What were the highlights of my day? What made me feel proud, happy, or grateful? These questions help you notice the positive moments that might otherwise be forgotten and encourage you to celebrate your efforts, even on challenging days.

Next, gently consider what was difficult or disappointing. Were there any moments when you felt stressed, frustrated, or discouraged? Did you face any setbacks or miss any goals? Instead of judging yourself harshly, treat these reflections as opportunities to learn. Ask yourself: What can I do differently tomorrow? How can I approach a similar situation with more patience, courage, or kindness? This mindset turns mistakes into stepping stones for future success.

A daily review is also a chance to reconnect with your intentions. Remind yourself of your bigger goals and values. Are your daily actions taking you in the direction you want to go? If not, what minor adjustments could you make? This regular check-in helps you stay aligned with what matters most, so you do not drift off course.

Writing your daily review in a journal can be especially helpful. You might jot down three things that went well, one challenge you faced, and one thing you want to try tomorrow. Over time, these daily entries create a record of your journey, showing how much you have learned and grown.

Some people like to add a short gratitude practice at the end of their review, listing one or two things they appreciate about the day. This small step trains your brain to look for the good, even during tough times, and builds a more positive, resilient mindset.

The power of the daily review comes from its consistency. By making it a habit—just a few minutes each evening—you give yourself the gift of self-awareness, learning, and motivation.

You become more attuned to your needs, strengths, and progress. Over weeks and months, the small lessons you gather each day add up, helping you handle challenges, celebrate victories, and keep moving forward.

A daily review is a simple tool, but its impact can be life-changing. With regular practice, you will feel more confident, clear-minded, and ready to make each day a step closer to your goals and dreams.

Turning Insights into Action

Reflection and self-discovery are valuable, but their true power is unlocked when you use your insights to create positive change in your life. Turning insights into action means taking what you have learned about yourself—your strengths, needs, values, and goals—and using that knowledge to make real improvements, one step at a time.

The first step is to notice which insights feel most important or inspiring. After journaling or reflecting, ask yourself: What stood out to me? Was there a new realization about a habit, a relationship, or a pattern in my thinking? You noticed you feel more confident when you set small goals, or you discovered that a particular routine helps you feel calm.

Next, choose one insight to focus on. Trying to change too much at once can be overwhelming, so start small. Decide on a specific action you can take based on what you have learned. For example, if you realize that morning walks help clear your mind, plan to set out your shoes the night before. If you know that you feel anxious in noisy environments, try using headphones or finding a quiet space for breaks.

Make your action step as clear and straightforward as possible. Instead of saying, "I will be healthier," try "I will pack a healthy lunch for work tomorrow." The more specific your action is, the easier it is to follow through.

It also helps to write your action steps down and set a reminder. Put it in your journal, on your calendar, or in your phone—somewhere you will see it. If your insight relates to a habit, set up your environment to support your new routine. Little changes, like leaving your journal on your pillow or keeping a gratitude list by your toothbrush, make it more likely that you'll take action.

Accountability can make a big difference. Share your insight and planned action with a friend, coach, or support group. Letting someone know what you are working on—and checking in with them about your progress—can help you stay motivated and committed.

Once you take your first action, pause to notice how it feels. Are you moving closer to your goal? What worked well, and what could be adjusted? Reflection is not a one-time process—it is a cycle. As you take action, keep checking in with yourself, learning, and adjusting as needed.

Growth is made up of small, steady steps. Even if things do not go perfectly, each effort brings you more self-awareness and closer to the life you want to build. Celebrate your progress, no matter how small. Each action you take based on your insights is a sign of your commitment to yourself and your future.

Turning insights into action, you transform self-reflection into real, lasting change. This practical approach helps you break old patterns, build new strengths, and create a more fulfilling, balanced life — one thoughtful step at a time.

CHAPTER 18

Purpose-Driven Living

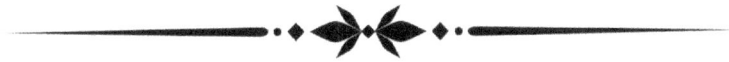

Living with purpose means having a sense of direction that guides your choices, fuels your motivation, and brings more profound meaning to your days. Purpose-driven living is about discovering what truly matters to you and allowing that sense of meaning to shape your actions, relationships, and dreams. In this chapter, you will explore how to find your unique sense of purpose, why it matters for happiness and resilience, and simple ways to live each day with intention and heart.

Discovering Your Life Purpose

Discovering your life purpose is a journey of self-exploration and curiosity. It is not about finding one big answer overnight, but about paying attention to the things that truly light you up and give your life meaning. Your purpose is personal; it is shaped by your values, interests, strengths, and the experiences that have moved you the most.

Start by reflecting on what makes you feel most alive. Think about the activities, conversations, or moments when you lose track of time because you are so engaged. What do you love to learn about, create, or share with others? These experiences often offer clues to what matters most to you.

Consider your strengths, the qualities or skills that come naturally or that others often notice in you. You may be a good listener, a creative thinker, a caring friend, or someone who brings energy to a group. Ask people you trust what they see as your unique gifts. Sometimes, those around us can see strengths we might overlook.

Another way to discover your purpose is to look at the challenges you have faced. Often, our most difficult experiences teach us essential lessons or spark a desire to help others in similar situations. For example, someone who struggled with loneliness might feel called to build community, while someone who overcame illness may want to inspire hope in others.

Ask yourself: What would I do if I knew I could not fail? What problems in the world do I wish I could help solve? What legacy do I want to leave behind? These questions allow you to see beyond everyday routines and focus on what truly matters.

Your purpose does not have to be grand or world-changing. It might be found in simple acts of kindness, raising a family, sharing art, or helping others grow. Purpose can change and evolve throughout your life as you grow and learn.

Discovering your life purpose is a process, not a destination. Stay open, curious, and compassionate with yourself as you explore. Over time, you will begin to see patterns and themes that point you toward the work, relationships, and experiences that make your life feel rich and meaningful.

Aligning Actions with Values

Once you start to understand what matters most to you, the next step is to make sure your daily actions match those values. Aligning your actions with your values is about living honestly, letting what you do reflect who you truly are inside. This can bring a deep sense of satisfaction, trust in yourself, and a feeling that your life is moving in the right direction.

Start by thinking about your core values. These are the beliefs or principles that guide you, such as kindness, honesty, creativity, family, health, growth, or service. You may value friendship and connection, or you may feel strongly about helping others, learning new things, or caring for the environment. Write down the values that feel most important to you, even just three to five to begin with.

Next, take a close look at how you spend your time and energy each day. Ask yourself: Do my actions reflect my values? For example, if you value health but rarely take time to rest or move your body, you might feel out of sync or dissatisfied. If you care about honesty but often hide your feelings to keep the peace, you might notice tension building up inside. These feelings are signals, gentle nudges that it is time to bring your actions and values closer together.

To align your actions with your values, choose one area of your life to focus on first. It might be your work, your relationships, your self-care, or how you spend your free time. Ask yourself, "What is one small step I can take this week to live more in line with what matters to me?" This could mean setting aside time for a favorite hobby, reaching out to someone you care about, or speaking up kindly but honestly when something matters to you.

It's normal to feel some discomfort at first, especially if you are used to putting others' needs before your own or following routines that no longer fit your values. Be gentle with yourself, real change happens one small action at a time. If you slip up, reflect on what happened and try again. Every effort to act in line with your values strengthens your sense of purpose and self-respect.

It may also be helpful to revisit your values from time to time. As you grow and change, your values shift, or new ones become more critical. Checking in with yourself helps you stay true to what matters most in each season of your life.

When your actions reflect your values, you are more likely to feel proud of your choices, build trust with others, and handle challenges with resilience and clarity. Even small steps taken with intention and heart can turn daily routines into a meaningful, purpose-driven life.

Creating a Personal Mission Statement

A personal mission statement is a simple yet powerful tool that helps guide your choices, actions, and goals. It is like a compass, a clear statement of what you stand for, what matters most to you, and the kind of person you want to be. Creating a personal mission statement can bring focus, motivation, and a more profound sense of purpose to your everyday life.

To start, spend some quiet time reflecting on your values, passions, and strengths. Think about what makes you feel alive, what you care about most, and the qualities you want to share with the world. Ask yourself:

- What values do I want to live by?
- What kind of impact do I want to have on others?
- What brings me meaning and joy?
- How do I want to grow and contribute, both personally and in my community?

Write down the words or phrases that come to mind. Do not worry about making it perfect, just let your thoughts flow. Sometimes, looking at examples can help. A mission statement might be as simple as:

"I aim to live each day with kindness, honesty, and courage, helping others and growing into my best self."

Or more specifically, like:

"My mission is to inspire hope, encourage learning, and build positive connections wherever I go."

It might focus on family, creativity, health, service, or any other area that feels meaningful to you.

Once you have a few ideas, start shaping your mission statement into one or two clear sentences. Keep it short, memorable, and accurate to you. Read it out loud, does it feel authentic? Does it excite or comfort you? Your mission statement should remind you of who you want to be, especially when you face choices or challenges.

After you've written your statement, place it somewhere you will see it often on your wall, in your journal, or as a reminder on your phone. Let it guide your decisions, big and small. When you are unsure about a direction, ask yourself, "Does this fit with my mission?" If not, consider what changes you might make.

Your mission statement can grow and change with you. Review it every few months or after significant life changes. Adjust it to fit your evolving dreams, values, and goals.

Creating a personal mission statement is not just a writing exercise; it is an act of self-leadership and care. It gives you a sense of direction and helps you live with more clarity, intention, and heart. By taking this step, you empower yourself to move forward in life guided by your unique sense of purpose.

Finding Meaning in Everyday Life

Meaning is not just found in significant achievements or life-changing moments; it can be discovered in the simple, ordinary parts of daily living. When you learn to notice and appreciate these small moments, life feels more prosperous, more joyful, and more connected to your sense of purpose.

One of the easiest ways to find meaning is to pay attention to the present moment. Whether you are making a cup of tea, caring for a loved one, or watching the sunrise, allow yourself to be fully there. Notice the sights, sounds, and feelings of the moment. Even the most routine tasks can become meaningful when you bring your awareness and care to them.

Acts of kindness, no matter how small, are another powerful source of meaning. Holding the door for someone, sharing a smile, or sending a message of encouragement can brighten your day and someone else's. These simple actions remind you that you make a difference, and they often create a ripple effect of positivity.

Relationships are a deep well of everyday meaning. Taking time to connect with family, friends, neighbors, or even strangers adds richness to life. Listening to someone, offering support, or sharing a laugh helps you feel seen and valued and gives you a chance to provide the same in return.

Meaning can also be found in growth and learning. Each time you try something new, overcome a challenge, or work toward a goal, you build confidence and discover new strengths. Even when things do not go perfectly, the effort you put in and the lessons you learn along the way give life more depth and purpose.

Expressing gratitude is a simple practice that brings more meaning into daily life. Please take a moment each day to notice what you appreciate, whether it's a favorite meal, a good conversation, or a peaceful walk. Keeping a gratitude journal or simply saying thank you, even silently, helps you focus on what is good and meaningful right now.

Personal rituals, no matter how small, can also give you a sense of structure and meaning. Whether it's morning coffee, an evening walk, or a weekly call with a friend, these routines create moments of comfort and reflection. They remind you that life is made up of many small experiences, each with its value.

Finding meaning in everyday life often comes from living in line with your values. When your actions reflect what matters most to you, kindness, honesty, creativity, or service, you naturally feel more fulfilled, even on ordinary days.

You do not need to wait for a big event to find meaning. It is always available, hidden in the details of each day. By slowing down, connecting, and living with intention, you turn everyday moments into sources of purpose, joy, and lasting satisfaction.

Serving Others as a Source of Strength

Serving others is one of the most meaningful ways to find strength, fulfillment, and purpose in your own life. While it might seem like helping others is only about giving, it gives back to you in countless ways. When you reach out, support someone in need, or make a positive difference, no matter how small, you often discover new energy, perspective, and a more profound sense of connection.

Service does not have to be grand or complicated. Sometimes, it is as simple as listening to a friend, helping a neighbor with groceries, volunteering a few hours a month, or offering encouragement to someone who is struggling. Every act of service, no matter the size, reminds you that you are part of a larger community and that your actions matter.

Helping others can be a powerful source of inner strength because it shifts your focus outward. When you are feeling low, anxious, or stuck, reaching out to help someone else can lift your mood and give you a new sense of purpose. Studies show that people who engage in acts of kindness or service experience less stress, greater happiness, and even improved physical health.

Serving others also builds resilience. When you support someone through a difficult time, you develop empathy and compassion not just for them, but for yourself as well. You begin to see that everyone faces challenges, and that by working together, you can overcome more than you ever could alone. This shared experience strengthens your sense of belonging and community.

Service often brings unexpected rewards. You might make new friends, learn new skills, or gain a fresh perspective on your own life. Sometimes, helping others allows you to see your strengths more clearly. You realize how much you have to offer, and you begin to feel more confident and hopeful about your journey.

If you are not sure where to start, look for simple ways to be of service in your everyday life. Offer a smile to a stranger, check in with someone who might be lonely, or look for local opportunities to volunteer your time or skills. Even small acts, such as holding a door, sharing a meal, or sending a thoughtful message, can have a significant impact.

Serving others is not about being perfect or giving until you are empty. It is about sharing what you can, when you can, and allowing those experiences to nourish your spirit. Service is a cycle; the more you give, the more you often receive in return.

Making service a regular part of your life, you build a strong foundation of inner strength, gratitude, and connection. In helping others, you allow yourself to grow, heal, and find deeper meaning every day.

CONCLUSION

Building inner strength is not a one-time task or a finish line you cross. It is a lifelong journey, a gentle, ongoing process of learning about yourself, facing challenges, and growing wiser and more resilient along the way. Your path will have smooth stretches and rocky patches, moments of joy and times of doubt. But with each step, you become stronger, more compassionate, and more true to who you are.

Inner strength comes from knowing and accepting yourself, flaws and all. It grows as you pay attention to your feelings, reflect on your experiences, and act in ways that match your values. This journey does not require perfection. Instead, it calls for honesty, curiosity, and a willingness to keep trying, even when things do not go as planned. Every challenge you face, every setback you overcome, adds another layer to your strength.

The lessons and tools you have explored in this book are not just ideas to read and set aside. They are invitations to action practices you can return to again and again, no matter where you are in life. Whether it is mindful self-reflection, journaling, gratitude, visualization, or serving others, each practice is a stepping stone that supports you on your path.

There will be times when you feel unsure or even lost. That is part of every meaningful journey. During those moments, remember that growth often happens quietly, beneath the surface, even when you cannot see it. Trust the process and permit yourself to rest when you need to. Inner strength includes the courage to pause, seek support, and ask for help.

You have learned that self-compassion is not a sign of weakness but a foundation for resilience. By treating yourself with kindness during hard times, you create the safety and stability needed to keep going. Allow yourself to celebrate your efforts, big and small, and forgive yourself when things do not work out. Each day is a new chance to begin again.

One of the most potent parts of building inner strength is the impact it has on others. When you show up authentically, support your loved ones, and give back to your community, you help create a world where everyone can feel stronger and more supported. Your actions, no matter how small, can inspire those around you and ripple outward in ways you may never fully see.

Remember, inner strength is not about never feeling afraid or struggling. It is about facing those feelings with courage, reaching out for connection, and believing in your ability to adapt and grow. It is about trusting that you have everything you need inside you to handle whatever comes your way.

As you continue your journey, keep your heart and mind open. Explore new practices, return to the ones that resonate most, and keep asking yourself what you need to feel balanced, hopeful, and alive. Let your values guide your choices, and be gentle with yourself on difficult days.

Surround yourself with supportive people who encourage your growth. Seek out mentors, friends, or communities who share your values and inspire you to keep moving forward. At the same time, learn to enjoy your own company and appreciate the strength that comes from within.

Your journey to inner strength will be uniquely yours, shaped by your dreams, challenges, relationships, and experiences. There is no single correct path, only the path that feels true for you. Be patient with yourself, and trust that you are always moving forward, even when progress feels slow.

As you close this book, take a moment to honor how far you have come. You have shown curiosity, courage, and care for your well-being. Carry these qualities with you as you continue growing and changing. Remember that every day brings new opportunities to practice inner strength, kindness, and purpose.

Your lifelong journey to inner strength is just that, a journey. It will continue to unfold, teaching you, challenging you, and helping you become the most authentic, resilient, and empowered version of yourself. Keep walking your path with hope, patience, and an open heart. The strength you build within will light the way, not just for you, but for everyone whose life you touch.